Ecological
Medicine

Ecological Medicine

Healing the Earth, Healing Ourselves

Edited by Kenny Ausubel
with J. P. Harpignies

Foreword by Andrew Weil, M.D.

Sierra Club Books
San Francisco

This book is intended as an informational guide. The remedies, techniques, and approaches described herein are meant to supplement, and not to be a substitute for, professional medical care or treatment. They should not be used to treat illness without prior consultation with a qualified health care professional.

The Sierra Club, founded in 1892 by John Muir, has devoted itself to the study and protection of the earth's scenic and ecological resources—mountains, wetlands, woodlands, wild shores and rivers, deserts and plains. The publishing program of the Sierra Club offers books to the public as a nonprofit educational service in the hope that they may enlarge the public's understanding of the Club's basic concerns. The point of view expressed in each book, however, does not necessarily represent that of the Club. The Sierra Club has some sixty chapters throughout the United States and in Canada. For information about how you may participate in its programs to preserve wilderness and the quality of life, please address inquiries to Sierra Club, 85 Second Street, San Francisco, California 94105, or visit our website at www.sierraclub.org.

"Hoxsey: When Healing Becomes a Crime" was published in slightly different form in *Tikkun* 16, no. 3 (May/June 2001). "The Coming Age of Ecological Medicine" was published in slightly different form in *Utne Reader*, no. 105 (May/June 2001).

Published by Sierra Club Books
85 Second Street, San Francisco, CA 94105
www.sierraclub.org/books

Produced and distributed by University of California Press
Berkeley and Los Angeles, California
University of California Press, Ltd.
London, England
www.ucpress.edu

SIERRA CLUB, SIERRA CLUB BOOKS, and the Sierra Club design logos are registered trademarks of the Sierra Club.

Library of Congress Cataloging-in-Publication Data

Ecological medicine : healing the earth, healing ourselves / edited by Kenny Ausubel with
    J. P. Harpignies; foreword by Andrew Weil.
        p. cm.
    Includes bibliographical references.
    ISBN 1-57805-098-7 (pbk. : alk. paper)
    1. Environmental health.   2. Ecology.   I. Ausubel, Ken.   II. Harpignies, J. P.

RA566.E25 2004
616.9'8—dc21   2003052808

Book and cover design by Lynne O'Neil
Printed in the United States of America on New Leaf Ecobook 50 acid-free paper, which contains a minimum of 50 percent post-consumer waste, processed chlorine free. Of the balance, 25 percent is Forest Stewardship Council certified to contain no old-growth trees and to be pulped totally chlorine free.

07 06 05 04   10 9 8 7 6 5 4 3 2 1

Contents

Foreword

YOU ARE ABOUT TO READ a collection of thoughtful essays on medicine and health—not just personal health but planetary health, and not just medicine in the ordinary sense but medicine as an enterprise that encompasses the totality of human experience. A unifying theme in these pages is reconnection with nature. All of the authors, myself included, feel that conventional science, medicine, and industry have separated us from nature, made us fearful of it, and encouraged us to try to control it in ways that have failed disastrously.

There is a sense of urgency in this writing, a sense that modern, urban, resource-gobbling, polluting civilization is about to reach its limit. In one way or another, its unhealthy relationship to nature will lead to inevitable failure, perhaps a very messy and catastrophic failure that will take a lot of us down with it. Things simply cannot keep going as they are.

If there is any chance of saving ourselves and the planet, it can only come from a change in consciousness. Although the root meaning of the word "medicine" is "thoughtful action to establish order," the word has become a synonym for physical remedies, especially drugs. This is in contrast to Native American usage, which emphasizes thoughtful action in the nonmaterial realm. Medicine men and medicine women are shamans, trained to mediate between the visible world of effects and the invisible world of causes. When Native Americans talk of "medicine" they are using the word in a much broader sense than most of us do.

We desperately need that larger kind of medicine if we are to avoid the catastrophe that looms before us. To manifest it we need the efforts of thought leaders and agents of change in our society. The contributors to this volume are such people, and the Bioneers Conference has provided a forum in which we can exchange ideas. The directions we must move in are clearly indicated in these pages, as are outlines of solutions to the problems we face. But the hour is late, and if ideas are to have power they must translate into action.

The most pessimistic experts tell us that even if we stopped everything we are doing that is leading to disaster, it would be too late; the momentum of our present course is so strong and its effects already so destructive that we cannot avoid certain doom. I do not share that attitude. Time and again in my medical practice I have experienced the power of healing. A change of consciousness that leads to thoughtful action can accomplish miracles. I hope that you, the reader, will be inspired by these words to act — in whatever way you can, in whatever sphere of influence you have— to bring the new medicine into being and to start the process of healing ourselves, our society, and our planet.

Andrew Weil, M.D.
Tucson, Arizona
February 2003

Acknowledgments

FIRST AND FOREMOST, I want to express my resounding gratitude and that of the Bioneers organization to the contributors to this book, who have so generously permitted us to feature their work here. We also thank them for their thoughtful review and enhancement of the material.

I offer my profound thanks to Dr. Andrew Weil for contributing the foreword and for his peerless vision in the field of ecological medicine.

In particular, I want to acknowledge two of the visionaries of ecological medicine who contributed to this book. Michael Lerner has been a paragon of leadership, compassion, and dedication whose pathfinding efforts have repeatedly expanded the vision of environmental health and grounded it in effective action. Carolyn Raffensperger has synthesized the essence of many fields and elegantly woven them together while purposefully advancing the precautionary principle, perhaps beyond what anyone thought possible.

The Bioneers and I are mightily grateful to Danny Moses, editor-in-chief of Sierra Club Books, who championed this project and gently and skillfully guided it to its full potential. I also offer my thanks to Jan Spauschus, whose thoughtful copyediting teased the book into more readable form.

The book would never have happened without the superlative contributions of several of my Bioneers colleagues: The incomparable J. P. Harpignies, my longtime collaborator and a central force in the Bioneers Conference since its inception, brought to a complex editing process his customary good humor, sage counsel, sophisticated perspectives, and frightening efficiency. To the introductions describing each contributor, he added his keen insight and singular capacity for cogently framing issues. Celeste DiFelici, the publications manager at Bioneers/CHI, has been an indefatigable associate, applying her sharp editorial intelligence and relentless attention to detail to the manuscript. Her can-do attitude and ability to keep a blur of balls in the air consistently uplifted both the book and the process. The amazing Nina Simons, executive director of Bioneers/CHI, gave her unwavering commitment to the project and integrated it effectively within the organizational ecology of the Bioneers. Bioneers managing director Ginny McGinn powered the project with a strong structure and support system, and her sure touch helped guide the project to completion. The unsinkable CHI coordinator Kelli Webster and Celeste DiFelici navigated a blizzard of transcriptions. Celeste and Amy Theobold pulled together the resources, gently nudging the contributors to provide their best lists.

To the Bioneers and the Collective Heritage Institute staff at large, endless appreciation and thanks for their cheerful and professional ongoing work of producing the annual Bioneers Conference, which is, after all, the wellspring of this book.

And last, many thanks to Nina Utne, Jay Walljasper, and Julie Ristau of *Utne Reader* for helping get the ball rolling by sifting ecological medicine out of the editorial pile and into the magazine, and for encouraging me to pursue this book from its conception.

Introduction

THIS BOOK LAUNCHES THE MAIDEN VOYAGE in a Bioneers series. Each volume in this anthology series will focus on a particular theme and will be drawn principally from the text of talks given by the rich array of contributors who speak at the annual Bioneers Conference.

As the first title in the series, *Ecological Medicine* reflects the essence of the cultural DNA encoded in Bioneers—biological pioneers. Ecological medicine is a unifying field that embodies the recognition that human and environmental health are inseparable. It is also a metaphor for the healing process intrinsic to life that applies to both ecosystems and our bodies. Environmental restoration is innately an enterprise of healing. This basic orientation of working with nature to help nature heal is the essence of the work of the Bioneers, who have peered deep into the heart of living systems to glean nature's own operating instructions.

I arrived at the threshold of ecological medicine through prior work in the realms of alternative medicine and the environment. Beginning in the early 1970s, I became closely involved in the nascent field of natural medicine as both a patient and a journalist. Having suffered a personal health crisis, I found conventional medicine unable to help me. I began exploring alternatives, not from any compelling philosophical bent, but out of the personal desperation of illness. I went on to become fascinated by the larger ideas embedded in a holistic medical approach, one that works with the body's own processes and strengthens its remarkable capacity for healing. That model stood in diametrical contrast to the standard "heroic" medical paradigm that discounts the body's own ability for self-repair and champions the physician's power to dominate, suppress, and kill disease.

In the course of my explorations, my father died suddenly of cancer at a relatively young age. This traumatic event shifted my attention to alternative cancer therapies, resulting in the film I produced in the 1980s on the once famous Hoxsey herbal cancer treatment (described later in this book). After being banned in the United States for political reasons, the treatment continues to be available at one lone clinic in Tijuana, Mexico. Streams of terminal cancer patients have had to cross an international border to obtain this harmless natural remedy. I decided to make the film partly in hopes of preventing this valuable treatment's eventual extinction.

While researching the botanical basis of the Hoxsey formulas, I met Gabriel Howearth, a master organic gardener and seed collector. He had been hired by San Juan Pueblo, an ancient Native American community in New Mexico, to help revive indigenous farming. He had planted dazzling gardens from the vast ark of traditional seeds he had collected throughout the Americas in an effort to conserve them. My experience at the pueblo was a revelatory and inspiring introduction to biodiversity in the garden and the wondrous fertility of natural farming.

I learned that these precious seeds, the genetic diversity that forms the very basis of global food security, were also under threat of extinction. Because these seeds could not be patented, giant seed companies, often owned by the same chemical and pharmaceutical conglomerates that opposed Hoxsey, were driving them from the marketplace. Gabriel and I decided to start a company, Seeds of Change, that would form a market partnership with backyard gardeners to help bring these irreplaceable seeds and foods back into the food web.

What struck me about both these projects was that they represented positive solutions to major problems: cancer and the loss of agricultural biodiversity. I had no illusions that they were panaceas that would by themselves overcome these huge challenges. But they seemed to me at least some part of a solution.

As both a journalist and concerned citizen, I decided to start poking around to see what other kinds of environmental solutions might exist. I began to encounter brilliant innovators who had devised effective approaches to the unfolding ecological crisis. The common thread was that they had looked to nature's own wisdom for guidance. I came to call them "Bioneers."

In 1990, I founded what became the Bioneers Conference to bring these brilliant social and scientific pathfinders together and to expose their highly practical work directly to the public. From the outset, one primary strand was green medicine, the rich panoply of therapeutic methods derived from natural sources or traditional and indigenous knowledge. In 1992, Dr. Andrew Weil, who can rightfully be called the godfather of ecological medicine, gave a luminous talk (reprinted here) portraying how medicine's separation from nature is at the root of many tragedies, both human and environmental.

In 1997, while writing a book on Hoxsey, I attended the first Comprehensive Cancer Care Conference, founded by Dr. James Gordon of the Center for Mind-Body Medicine. The event was a landmark gathering that brought together many of the leading lights of alternative cancer therapy with conventional practitioners and cancer patients. It came at a seminal moment when alternative medicine was unequivocally going mainstream. Everyone there recognized that the conference signaled a profound and irrevocable shift in medical practice and philosophy.

Yet as I listened to speaker after brilliant speaker, I found myself deeply troubled. Out of forty presenters discussing cancer, only two even mentioned the environment. How could such a basic disconnection occur? After all, cancer is the very metaphor of industrial civilization, the deadly shadow that is an unmistakable indicator that something has gone terribly wrong. How could medicine so woefully neglect the overwhelmingly environmental roots of this dreaded global pandemic?

Having one foot in the worlds of both alternative medicine and the environment, I wondered why these two crucial and interrelated communities had evolved so separately and were still barely talking to each other. I decided in that moment to use the Bioneers as a platform to help bridge the gap between them. The 1999 conference highlighted the emerging environmental health movement and featured a clarion call (reprinted here) by Michael Lerner, a longstanding visionary in the field.

Around that time, I had the good fortune to connect with Carolyn Raffensperger, whose work had increasingly focused on the precautionary principle. One day she sent me some chicken-scratch notes on ideas she was noodling around with. She laid out the bones of something she called "ecological medicine," succinctly framing the essential convergence of human health and the environment. She pointed the way to a medicine that resides in the natural world and that positions human health as dependent on the larger condition of ecological health. Our interaction resulted in "The Coming Age of Ecological Medicine," an article I wrote for *Utne Reader* (reprinted here) surveying the terrain of this budding movement. Since that time, a vibrant network has begun to form that advances the ideas and practices of ecological medicine.

For many people, a personal health crisis is often the doorway into environmental awareness. We are compelled to look at what we eat and how that food was grown and made. We begin to look into possible exposures to poisons and chemicals in our immediate environment or workplace. We question whether the "side effects" of the drugs or technological interventions offered us by the medical profession are worth the price our bodies will pay. We come to realize that none of us is immune to the assault of environmental harms compromising our health and that we cannot ultimately solve our personal health problems without cleaning up the environment. We have to wonder what kind of world we are giving our children and how we can better protect their health and well-being. We search out tangible answers and solutions, building on the successful models of others.

The good news is that for the most part the answers to our problems are present. A vibrant culture of innovative solutions is being born out of this cataclysm and it's spreading. The models percolate up from the deep wisdom of the natural world. Extraordinary human creativity focused on problem solving is exploding the mythology of despair. Together these solutions and models point to a Declaration of Interdependence.

Ecology is the elegant art of relationships in the fantastically elaborate web of life. As in quantum physics, it's a world not primarily of things but of relationships. While disruptions to ecosystems can engender cascades of negative repercussions, there are complementary sets of beneficial feedback loops. Ecological restoration sets in motion synergistic dynamics that promote stability and health. We can contribute positively to that process by cultivating and honoring life's intricate, idiosyncratic tapestry, navigating by the evolutionary north star of symbiosis. As biomimicry researcher Janine Benyus has cogently put it, "What life does is to create conditions conducive to life."

The great health advances of the nineteenth century had little to do with medical care and everything to do with strategic public health measures. Diseases were dramatically controlled by a collection of societal changes, such as maintaining clean water supplies and quarantining the sick. The result was a steep decline in diseases, including tuberculosis, cholera, and diphtheria, before there were drugs to treat these illnesses or vaccines to prevent them.

In the later nineteenth century, there raged a fundamental conflict of medical opinion between Louis Pasteur and his scientific rival Antoine Béchamp. Whereas Pasteur identified pathogenic germs as the cause of disease, Béchamp contended that "the terrain is everything." In his view, it is principally an imbalance in the body's own ecology that allows dangerous germs to gain dominance or stimulates otherwise harmless germs to mutate and become malignant. A healthy "terrain," he proposed, defeats pathogens or holds them in check in a subtle dynamic balance.

In other words, to borrow Marshall McLuhan's phrase, the medium is the message in biology, too.

Ecological medicine shifts the emphasis from the individual to public health; from nutrition to the food web and farming systems; from a human-centered viewpoint to one of biodiversity and all the other ecosystem services that are the foundations of health and healthy economies. It is founded in the precautionary principle, and it calls for a new social contract with both the human family and the web of life.

We hope this book will shed light on what some of the best and brightest have begun to figure out. Because it is an anthology derived from talks at the Bioneers Conference, it is not comprehensive or encyclopedic, and doesn't pretend to cover everything in this vast field. (Some topics not covered here will be addressed in future books.)

The many brilliant contributors represented in these pages celebrate the reconsecration of the human-nature relationship in a joyous marriage. They honor the genius of nature, which offers us the solutions we so urgently need today to heal both ourselves and the planet that is our home and home to many others.

Speaking at the Bioneers Conference, author Frances Moore Lappé once probed the question of how societies undergo fundamental change. She had studied why it was that Europe finally abandoned the divine right of monarchies. Her conclusion was simple: People just stopped believing in it.

Ideas can be more powerful than even entrenched economic and political systems. Ecological medicine is an idea whose time has come, and it is unstoppable.

> Kenny Ausubel
> Santa Fe, New Mexico
> February 2003

Part I

Ecological Medicine:
One Notion, Indivisible

The Coming Age
of Ecological Medicine

Kenny Ausubel

AMONG THE MANY IMMIGRANTS who arrived in New York City
in the summer of 1999, none made a name for itself more quickly than West
Nile virus. Traced to a virus spread by mosquitoes, the disease had never been
seen in this country, or even in the western hemisphere. It first struck birds,
then people, killing seven and sickening dozens more. The city hoped to control it by killing the mosquitoes with malathion, a pesticide chemically related
to nerve gas. Though many protested, Mayor Rudolph Giuliani insisted the
spraying was perfectly safe.

Within months, scientists at the U.S. Environmental Protection Agency
(EPA) were debating just how wrong the mayor had been. The EPA was on
the verge of declaring malathion a "likely" human carcinogen when its manufacturer protested. The EPA backed off, saying malathion posed no documented threat, though some in the agency continued to insist the dangers were
being downplayed. More suspicion was raised upon news of a massive die-
off of lobsters in Long Island Sound, near New York City. Malathion is known
to kill lobsters and other marine life, but officials denied the connection.

Though no direct causal link can yet be drawn, some infectious-disease
experts say anomalous outbreaks such as that of West Nile may be tied to human impacts on the environment, which have resulted in climate change and
the destruction of natural habitats. Dr. Paul R. Epstein, associate director of
the Center for Health and the Global Environment at Harvard Medical
School, has noted, "West Nile is getting veterinarians and doctors and biologists to sit down at the same table." What they are unraveling is a complex
knot linking human health and the state of the natural world.

3

Welcome to a preview of the health issues awaiting us in the twenty-first century. Indeed, we're already living at a time when vast social and biological forces are interacting in complex ways—and with unpredictable results. War, famine, and ecological damage have caused great human dislocations, which in turn have transformed tuberculosis, AIDS, and other modern plagues into global pandemics. Even more disturbing, many of our efforts to fight disease today are themselves symptoms of a deeper illness. Spraying an urban area with a substance whose health effects remain unknown is one glaring example, but there are many others. Think of certain compounds used in chemotherapy that more often kill than cure. Or the 100,000 people who die in hospitals every year from drugs that are properly prescribed. Or the many IV bags and other plastic medical products that release dioxin into the air when they are burned. That last example contributes to perhaps the most heartbreaking metaphor for our environmental abuse and its unforeseen consequences—the discovery that a human mother's milk is among the most toxic human foods, laced with dioxin, a confirmed carcinogen, and other chemical contaminants. All of these cases suggest our culture's deep dependence on synthetic chemicals and our long refusal to acknowledge how profoundly these have disrupted our ecological systems.

There's a widespread sense that mainstream medicine is blind to this reality and is even part of the problem. Growing disillusion over this, coupled with the fact that high-tech medicine costs too much and often doesn't work, has led to a widespread public search for alternatives. One result is the rise of complementary medicine, which combines the best of modern health care with other approaches. Add the immense new interest in traditional healing methods, herbs, and other natural remedies, and you get a sense of how much the health care paradigm has changed over the past thirty years.

What I see happening is a deeper shift that all of these approaches are edging us toward, even if we don't fully realize it yet. It's a new understanding of health and illness that has begun to move away from treating only the individual. Instead, good health lies in recognizing that each of us is part of a wider web of life. When the web is healthy, we are more likely to be healthy. But the environmental illnesses we see more and more of these days—rising cancer rates spring to mind—are constant reminders that the web is not healthy. How did we reach this tragic place? And more to the point, where do we go from here?

The first step toward a healthier future, I believe, lies in ecological medicine. Pioneered by a global movement of concerned scientists, doctors, and many others, ecological medicine is a loosely shared philosophy based on advancing public health by improving the environment. Its central idea is that industrial civilization has made a basic error in acting as if humans were apart from, rather than a part of, nature. Just as the knee bone is connected to the thigh bone, human and environmental health are inseparable. And in a biosphere that is rampantly toxic and woefully depleted, a mounting number of our health problems can only be understood as part of a larger pattern. Ecological medicine could well emerge as a force for dramatic cultural change. It proposes to reshape how industrial civilization operates, in part by redefining the role that the public plays in making the decisions that affect all life on earth.

Simply stated, improving human health is inextricably linked to restoring ecological well-being. The interconnectedness of all life is a fundamental biological truth. What's more, all life is under threat. There simply is no "elsewhere" to dump the hazardous by-products of industrial society. Eliminating them from our production systems is the only real solution, and a well-informed public is absolutely crucial to realizing it. In the words of Carolyn Raffensperger, executive director of the Science and Environmental Health Network (SEHN), a "truly holistic medicine extends beyond the mind-body connection to the human-planet whole." Here are some basic tenets of ecological medicine:

- The first goal of medicine is to establish the conditions for health and wholeness, thus preventing disease and illness. The second goal is to cure.

- The earth is also the physician's client. The patient under the physician's care is one part of the earth.

- Humans are part of a local ecosystem. Following the ecopsychological insight that a disturbed ecosystem can make people mentally ill, a disturbed ecosystem can surely make people physically ill.

• Medicine should not add to the illnesses of humans or the planet. Medical practices themselves should not damage other species or the ecosystem.

The main tool for putting these ideals into practice, ecological healers say, is what they call the precautionary principle. As articulated by Raffensperger and others, the precautionary principle basically argues that science and industry must fully assess the impact of their activities before they impose them upon the public and the environment. Societies around the world have begun to incorporate some version of the principle into law, hoping to rein in bioengineering and other new technologies. That science should objectively prove the safety of its own inventions might seem like common sense, but that's not how most science operates today.

For decades, the scientific and medical communities have operated on the principle that a certain amount of pollution and disease is the price we have to pay for modern life. This is called the risk paradigm, and it essentially means that it is society's burden to prove that new technologies and industrial processes are harmful, usually one chemical or technology at a time. The risk paradigm assumes that there are "acceptable" levels of contamination that the earth and our bodies can assimilate. It also allows a small, self-interested elite to set these levels, undistracted by the "irrational" fears and demands of the public. The "science" behind it is driven by large commercial interests and can hardly be considered impartial or in the public interest. Viewed with any distance at all, the risk paradigm is at best a high-stakes game of biological roulette with all the chambers loaded.

There is a global effort afoot today to replace the risk paradigm with the precautionary principle, which is based on a recognition that the ability of science to predict consequences and possible harm is limited. The precautionary principle acknowledges that all life is interconnected. It shifts the burden of proof (and liability) to the parties promoting potentially harmful technologies, and it limits the use of those technologies to experiments until they are proven truly safe.

The idea is not new—a version of it first appeared in U.S. law back in 1958 in the Delaney Amendment, which governed pesticide residues in food and set standards for environmental impact statements—nor is it radical. At its essence, the principle harks back to grandma's admonitions that "an ounce of prevention is worth a pound of cure" and that we're "better safe than sorry." The model is already used, in theory, for the drug industry, which is legally bound to prove drugs safe and effective prior to their use. Critics call it anti-scientific; they say it limits trade and stifles innovation. Advocates disagree.

"The precautionary principle actually shines a bright light on science," says Dr. Ted Schettler, science director of SEHN. "It doesn't tell us what to do, but it does tell you what to look at." Germany and Sweden have incorporated the principle into certain environmental policies. The United Nations Biosafety Protocol includes it in new guidelines for regulating trade in genetically modified products, its first appearance in an international treaty.

As people and their governments face ever more complex scientific decisions, the precautionary principle can serve as what some have called an insurance policy against our own ignorance. After all, we can't predict next week's weather or the economy a year out, much less the unfathomable complexity of living systems.

The Greek physician Hippocrates urged doctors to "do no harm," yet our medical practices often pose serious environmental threats. In 1994, for instance, the EPA reported that medical waste incinerators were the biggest source of dioxin air pollution in the United States. Dioxin finds its way into our food and accumulates in our fat; it's been linked to neurological damage in fetuses. Even a simple thermometer contains mercury, another potentially deadly neurotoxin.

The medical waste problem does not stop there. Along with generating radioactive waste from X rays and other treatments, the medical industry is now the source of a new peril: pharmaceutical pollution. Creatures living in lakes and rivers appear to be at special risk as antibiotics, estrogen, birth control pills, painkillers, and other drugs find their way into the waste stream. Fish are already affected; intersex mutations (in which the fish show both male and female characteristics) have been reported in various species around the world. And humans are not immune. The war on drugs may soon take on a new meaning as entire populations are subjected to constant low doses of pharmaceuticals in the water supply.

Groups like Health Care without Harm (www.noharm.org) have made it their mission to halt or curb such damaging medical practices, especially the use of mercury thermometers and the industry's reliance on burning its waste. Health Care without Harm, with 423 member organizations in 51 countries, has made great strides in this area, in part by directly confronting companies that engage in environmentally harmful practices. Another group, Greater Boston Physicians for Social Responsibility, has published a report with the Clean Water Fund, "In Harm's Way," that documents the many toxic threats to child development (http://psr.igc.org/ihw.htm).

Ecological medicine suggests first doing no harm to the environment, then going further, creating a medical practice that itself minimizes harm. Like virtually all earlier healing traditions, it emphasizes prevention, strengthening the organism and the environment to avoid illness in the first place. (Ancient Chinese healers, for instance, expected compensation only if their clients remained well, not if they got sick.)

But an ecological approach to healing also looks to deeper tenets embedded in nature itself and how it operates. Again, the new vision reveals itself to be in many ways an old one. It borrows from the insights of indigenous healing traditions, many of which are now being confirmed by modern science—including the fact that nature has an extraordinary and mysterious capacity for self-repair.

However resilient the biosphere may be, it's crucial to understand that the planet's basic life support systems are in serious decline. From climate change to plummeting biodiversity to gargantuan quantities of toxic wastes, ecological stresses are reaching dangerous thresholds. Much of the damage can be traced to the twentieth century's three most destructive technologies:

- Apart from helping induce potentially cataclysmic climate change, the *petrochemical industry* has unleashed 80,000 or so synthetic compounds that now permeate our land, water, and air, as well as our bodies. While some may be benign, the truth is that most have never been tested adequately enough to ascertain their safety—and even fewer have been measured for their cumulative effects on people and the environment or how they interact with other chemicals as they occur in real life.

- *Nuclear energy* use has led to the spread of radioactivity and virtually indestructible toxic-waste products into living systems worldwide. While public dread may focus on catastrophic accidents like the Chernobyl meltdown in 1986, other ill effects may come from steady exposure to low levels of radiation.

- *Genetic engineering* is introducing biological pollution that literally has a life of its own, a gene genie that cannot be put back in the bottle.

In addition to instructing healers first to do no harm, Hippocrates counseled physicians to "revere the healing force of nature." For years, that's been my quest: to work with nature to help nature heal. I founded the Bioneers Conference in 1990 to bring together people exploring ways of doing this— biological pioneers from many cultures and disciplines, and from all walks of life. All had peered deep into the heart of the earth's own living systems to understand what we can learn from 3.8 billion years of evolution. Their common purpose was to heal the earth. Their basic question: How would nature do it? They were using their knowledge of living systems to devise solutions to our most pressing environmental and societal problems. These people are modern healers too.

As their work repeatedly illustrates, many of the technologies we need to retool our industrial system already exist. Many of the Bioneers show how we can replace existing industrial practices with sustainable alternatives that run on clean, renewable energy sources and eliminate toxic emissions. Government has a role to play in this process too. Several years ago Sweden imposed a steep tax on pesticides, a measure that greatly reduced their use. Europe recently banned four antibiotics from animal feed. On the other side of the equation, governments are looking to promote tax subsidies for benign alternative technologies such as chlorine-free paper production and organic farming. (The city of Munich pays German farmers to grow organically in the watershed that supplies the city's drinking water.)

The ecological medicine movement proposes to green the practices of the health care industry and help mainstream medicine become safer.

The ethic of preventing harm that prevails in both environmental protection and ecological medicine will continue to spread, but what about existing messes? Many treatment methods modeled on living systems have shown dramatic capacities for bioremediation—that is, for detoxifying land, air, and water, Visionary biologist John Todd's "living machines" mimic natural ecologies by utilizing bacteria, fungi, plants, fish, and mammals to purify water and industrial wastes. The work of mycologist Paul Stamets has shown that fungi can help digest diesel spills and even chemical and biological weapons components. Similar success stories are found across many fields. By looking to the principles of ecological healing to restore the earth and ourselves, we create not only the conditions for individual health but also the basis for healthy societies and robust economies.

Biology is not rocket science. Rather, it is the superb art of relationships in the fantastically complex web of life. By mimicking nature, these approaches foster the healing that is the essence of living systems. Consider again the relationship between a nursing mother and her child. Despite the toxins that are now found in mothers' milk, it is still the best food for babies. Children fed breast milk are healthier because it confers immunity and unmatched nutrition. Which brings us back to the essence of ecological healing: In the wisdom of nature also lies the solution.

Alternative medicine is arguably the single largest progressive social movement of our era. As it becomes ever more mainstream, those working to advance public health are increasingly collaborating with those working to restore the earth's ecological health. Growing public awareness of the direct links between our personal health and environmental health is arising as a potent force in global politics. As suggested by Michael Lerner, founder of Commonweal, environmental health could well emerge as the central human rights issue of our age. We all have the right to be born free—free from poisons.

As human beings, we have a remarkable ability to reinvent our societies very rapidly. Our task now is to create an earth-honoring culture founded in the sanctity of life and the sacred human-nature relationship. Along with many others, I herald for this new century a Declaration of Interdependence flowing from the simple recognition that all life is connected. At its heart is ecological medicine, teaching us that we are the land and water and air. By restoring the earth, we restore ourselves.

Personal Healing
and Planetary Healing

Michael Lerner

It would be difficult to overstate the contributions Michael Lerner has made to the environmental health movement. He has been a guiding light who has brought his unblinking honesty, fairness, and compassion to bear on everything from the briar patch of alternative cancer therapies to the sinkhole of the human health effects of toxics.

He is the president and cofounder of Commonweal, the respected health and environmental research institute and think tank in Bolinas, California. He is cofounder of the Commonweal Cancer Help Program, whose groundbreaking approach was featured in Bill Moyers's historic Healing and the Mind *television series. He is the author of the classic book* Choices in Healing: Integrating the Best of Conventional and Complementary Approaches to Cancer, *as well as the winner of a MacArthur Fellowship, among many other honors.*

Michael was instrumental in helping launch Health Care without Harm, a seminal organization that first grew out of a conference held at Commonweal in 1996. It's an inspiring coalition of groups that conducts highly focused campaigns to stop the environmental and human health harms created by medicine itself. It has served as a prototype for the kinds of alliances necessary to reverse the poisoning of our ecosystems, our bodies, and our future and to bring about a health care system that truly "does no harm." He has helped envision powerful, effective new alliances among sectors of the alternative medicine movement, mainstream medical practitioners, workers, patients and patient advocates, and the environmental community to demand a nontoxic industrial revolution. He is currently engaged in building the Collaborative on Health and the Environment, a national partnership of organizations and individuals committed to protecting our health and preserving the environment.

❀   ❀   ❀

I COME FROM A LITTLE health and environmental center called Commonweal where for the last twenty-five years we have worked with kids with learning and behavior disorders and with adults with cancer. My colleague, Rachel Naomi Remmen, works with physicians who treat people with life-threatening illnesses, and we also address global environmental issues.

Health Care without Harm started at Commonweal with thirty citizen activists, scientists, and health-affected people who decided that of all the different forms of contamination we're witnessing, the fact that hospitals were a leading source of dioxin and mercury exposure for the American people just didn't make a lot of sense.

Health Care without Harm has now grown to approximately 423 organizations in 51 countries. It has closed down hundreds of medical waste incinerators worldwide and prevented the placement of hundreds more in poor communities. It is leading the effort to ban or phase out mercury thermometers in the United States and around the world. The mercury thermometer is interesting, because although health care only accounts for a small amount of total mercury exposure, everybody has that mercury thermometer in the bathroom. The act of asking yourself how to dispose of this mercury thermometer, realizing that this mercury can contaminate a twenty-acre lake, can help you realize that our coal plants and other major sources of mercury need really serious attention.

Health Care without Harm and the Commonweal Cancer Help Program have been the two really transformative experiences of the last fifteen years for me. For ninety-six weeks I've lived with people with cancer at Commonweal, small groups that are there doing yoga, meditation, imagery, and group support, eating a vegetarian diet and receiving massage. Most of them are women with breast cancer; many of them are young women with metastatic breast cancer and small children.

I want to tell you the story of one of these young women. She came to our Smith Farm Cancer Help Program in Washington, D.C. She was thirty-two years old, she was married to a carpenter, she had a three-year-old son and an eighteen-month-old daughter, and she had metastatic breast cancer that was moving very rapidly. On one evening, we talk about death and dying, about how to die as well as possible when that time comes. There are a lot of choices, and in the face of the anxiety and fear that people often bring into the program, the evening on death and dying is often liberating.

This young woman sat through the evening listening and taking some notes. At the end, as other people got up and began to move around to get tea or coffee, she sat in her chair. I noticed that she had begun to sort of shake and spasm. So I walked over to her with Jnani Chapman, who is our lead massage person on the program. As we got closer to her, we thought she was having an epileptic seizure of some kind, so we both instinctively began to hold her. I was holding her shoulders and Jnani was holding her legs.

Then I began to realize this wasn't an epileptic seizure; this was the totality of sadness and despair that this young woman was carrying. No matter what we said about how you could die well, the fact that she was, in her early thirties and with two very young children, going to have to die of breast cancer was just too overwhelming to take. So we sat with her and we held her as she went through these spasms and into sobbing, until finally it diminished. For me she is a very vivid reminder that no matter how well we learn to die, no matter how spiritual we are, whatever that means—and it can mean a lot— we're living in an epidemic of breast cancer. Not only breast cancer, but many other forms of cancer, and not only cancer, but learning disabilities, behavior disorders, endometriosis, infertility, and a wide range of chronic health problems that are related to chemical exposures and other environmental realities.

There is a new analysis emerging that we are living in an age of extinctions. But we are also witnessing an emerging environmental health movement that is a great source of hope in the face of what we are doing to the earth. Scientists are very clear that we are living in an age in which we are driving biodiversity—the sacred tree of life—back sixty-five million years, to its lowest level of vitality since the end of the age of the dinosaurs. This is the sixth great spasm of extinctions in the history of the earth, and it's being caused by human beings.

There are four great drivers of this age of extinctions: climate change, ozone depletion, toxic chemicals, and habitat destruction. We could speak at length of each. We could speak of climate change: We face droughts, floods, hurricanes, crop failures, melting polar ice caps, tens of millions of environmental refugees, island nations at risk of submersion. We could talk about ozone depletion: Rates of malignant melanoma and depleted immune systems are rising as a result of radiation exposure. We could talk about habitat destruction: The forests, the lungs of the earth, are being destroyed, and "new" viruses such as HIV and other extant and potential modern plagues are leaping from species to species in disrupted habitats.

I'm going to focus on chemicals, because this is one issue with which we have a very intimate relationship: These chemicals are in our bodies. There's a great book called *Our Stolen Future*, by Theo Colborn, Dianne Dumanoski, and John Peterson Myers, that has spawned a whole new literature on endocrine-disrupting chemicals. Endocrine disruption is something that happens to the developing fetus in the womb. The fetus is exquisitely vulnerable to these chemicals because they mimic the signals that the mother's endocrine system sends to the fetus to guide its development.

At infinitely lower levels than those at which chemicals cause cancer, at parts per billion or parts per trillion, these chemicals can shape the development of the fetus and cause a wide array of impacts on health, fertility, and intelligence. The simple truth is that we are now all holding body burdens of these chemicals that are comparable to those at which we see demonstrable health effects on wildlife and in laboratory animals. The results are links—not yet easy to make, but growing in strength—to breast cancer, testicular cancer, learning disabilities, behavior disorders, endometriosis, infertility, precocious puberty, shifting sex ratios, and neurological conditions.

In animal research, we see that there are changes in gender orientation in wildlife around the Great Lakes. In Florida, the alligators with the famous micro-penises are a result of chemical exposures. One percent of polar bears on an island in the Arctic have dual sex organs as a result of chemical exposures. The list goes on. Babies of mothers who eat a lot of Great Lakes fish with high chemical loads startle easily, are hard to console, and have learning and behavior disorders in school.

A new assessment confirms that sperm counts are declining in the industrial world. Another study shows two ubiquitous endocrine disrupters have estrogenic impacts on mice at concentrations comparable to those present in many people. A study by the Learning Disabilities Association analyzes the chemical pollutants that affect child development in learning in the United States. Twenty-four billion pounds of developmental toxicants are released in the United States annually, and 17 percent of kids have developmental learning or behavior disorders. Levels of the endocrine-disrupting chemicals called phthalates are very high in women of childbearing age, and they probably come from hair sprays, nail polishes, and perfumes. A recent report disclosed that girls in Puerto Rico with early breast development had seven times the level of the phthalate DEHP that girls with normal breast development had.

Another report found that brominated flame retardants, which interfere with thyroid function and can drastically affect mental competency, are being found in breast milk. Low levels of dioxin (which results from burning the PVC plastics in medical waste) interfere with vaginal development in rats. Children born to women who experienced early puberty—remember, we just linked that to chemicals—are more likely to develop asthma and allergies.

These reports go on and on and on, and I want to give you one image which to me encapsulates all of them. It's a tragic image, and I'm sorry to have to discuss it, but I believe it's important because it's the kind of thing that mobilizes people: Human breast milk has become one of the most toxic foods. The higher you live and eat on the food chain, the more toxins are concentrated in your body. Toxin levels increase fifty- or a hundredfold with every step up the food chain. Humans live near the top of the food chain, and babies drinking breast milk are one level higher. In fact, the only known way to reduce the level of toxic chemicals in your body is to get pregnant and breastfeed your first baby: A mother's level of persistent organic pollutants declines very significantly when she gives them to her baby, who then carries that as part of her lifetime body burden.

When I think of that young mother dying prematurely of breast cancer, when I think of the fact that the breasts of women have become toxic waste dumps—it's just not acceptable. It's important to state that breast milk is still the best food for babies. In spite of the toxic chemicals, kids fed breast milk do better than kids who get formula, because the main damage has been done in the womb, in fetal development. The positive benefits of breast-feeding still far outweigh those of feeding formula. But it's just not acceptable that we are putting women in a situation where they have to make choices of that kind.

However, I think it's very important not to see this situation as hopeless. I love the quote from Vaclav Havel, the great Czech statesman and playwright, who distinguished between optimism and hope. "Optimism," he said, "is the belief that everything is going to go right." But hope is very different. "Hope," he said, "is a deep orientation of the human soul that can be held in the darkest of times." On the one hand, these are affluent times; on the other, these are dark times for life on earth.

If we ask ourselves where we can find true hope, it is instructive to look back over the last few hundred years of human history. What was it like for the early activists who tried to replace monarchies with democracies? What was it like for the early Quakers who thought that they might end slavery? What was it like for Florence Nightingale and all those in the nineteenth century who literally transformed the world when they began to understand that infectious disease vectors could be changed by public health measures (which is a very important example of what we need to do)? In our own time, we've seen the labor movement, the civil rights movement, the peace movement, the environmental movement, the women's rights movement, the anti-apartheid movement, and the gay rights movement. These collective shifts in consciousness are very, very important.

I believe that we are now witnessing such a shift with regard to environmental health. Health Care without Harm is a model of a new kind of very smart, grassroots-based, market-focused campaign that isn't aimed so much at changing government regulations as at changing corporate behavior in the marketplace.

It has worked by creating very, very wide coalitions. You focus on a single narrow point that everybody agrees on, like the fact that dioxin and mercury shouldn't be coming out of hospitals, and then you work with these corporations, because hospitals, like other corporations, want to have a good name. You say, "Gee, wouldn't you like to make this little change, which you can make and we can show you the way, instead of having this very wide coalition, not only of environmentalists but of labor, faith-based groups, health-affected groups, and so on, all concerned with your behavior?"

These campaigns—Internet-based, market-focused, grassroots, wide coalitions—are changing the face of activism across the world. It's happening not only in health care but in the building industry (with green buildings), in the auto industry, in computers, schools, sustainable agriculture, and the military. Sector by sector, we're organizing innovative campaigns that focus on changing corporate behavior.

A whole new analytic synthesis is coalescing around issues of globalization, human rights, women's rights, the environment, corporate power and accountability, environmental justice, the unfinished agenda of race, the responsibilities of faith communities, and the question of who owns science. Toxicology is largely owned by the chemical corporations, and we can't have science owned by corporations. If science is owned by corporations, and the media are owned by corporations, we do not have the feedback loops that we need.

We have to turn that dynamic around. Democracy is not real unless we do. The great Buddhist educator and peace activist Thich Nhat Hanh said that we need to move to an age of what he calls Interbeing—an age of awareness that life is truly one. When medical waste incinerators in the United States are poisoning the Inuit people in the Arctic Circle and creating chemicals that every single baby around the world is born with and that are in the breast milk of every mother, we are all one. And we are one with the dolphins and whales and seals that are carrying these chemicals. The oneness of life is being brought back to us with a power and a literalness that we can no longer escape, and that awareness of Interbeing is what is fueling this emerging environmental health movement.

I believe that we are the ones who are destined to do this work. We really don't have any choice. The question is not so much whether we are going to win or lose this war, because we can't really control that. We don't know whether the powers of destruction are going to turn out to be greater in our time than the powers of life. But I would encourage each of you, no matter where you find yourself, no matter what field you're involved in, to begin to recognize that it's not a question of whether we win or lose. Hopelessness is not a very interesting way to live, and activism, engagement—however we do it—holding that vision, holding that hope in this darkest of times, is a form of witness, and it's the most interesting way to live.

Thinking Like a Girl
Is Good Medicine

Charlotte Brody

When it comes to environmental health, Charlotte Brody gets that particular Chesire cat smile that tells you she suspects you'll be won over to her impeccably conceived conclusions once you know what she knows. But more than that, she retains an authentic openness to the viewpoints of others, which probably explains why she has been so effective in starting to bring ecological medicine into mainstream medicine.

She began as a registered nurse and went on to become the coordinator of the Carolina Brown Lung Association, the director of a Planned Parenthood affiliate in North Carolina, and the organizing director of the Center for Health, Environment and Justice. Then, already a leading figure in the grassroots environmental movement, she cofounded Health Care without Harm, where she currently serves as co—executive director. The group, one of the most effective and innovative coalitions in the world today, has been a lighthouse in the environmental health movement, illuminating the tragic irony that the health care industry itself generates a litany of toxic harms.

Health Care without Harm reflects Charlotte's comprehensive and holistic approach. It has been unique in building broad coalitions of health care professionals, unions and workers, environmentalists, and citizens' groups to reduce and ultimately stop the release of toxics by the medical industry, while raising global awareness of the risks of toxics in the environment. Among its most recent successes was the national "Not Too Pretty" campaign that Charlotte helped conceive and manage to highlight the use of phthalates and other chemicals in beauty products marketed to women of childbearing age that may induce birth defects. The campaign sent floods of e-mails to the Food and Drug Administration (FDA) from thousands of women protest-ing the agency's neglect of this "Not Too Pretty" picture.

                                    ❀   ❀   ❀

HEALTH CARE WITHOUT HARM is a coalition working to provide practical solutions to the irony that health care practices themselves often make the environment—and people as part of the environment—sick.

Health Care without Harm members have closed down incinerators that pollute the environment and pollute all of us with dioxin and mercury. When we started, the U.S. EPA estimated that there were about 6,000 medical waste incinerators in the United States, and their most recent estimates say that there are fewer than 800. In the Philippines we've worked to get a ban on the in-cineration of medical and other toxic waste. Health Care without Harm has worked to end the use of mercury-containing medical devices, both by get-ting over 1,000 hospitals and health care systems to pledge to phase out the use of mercury in thermometers, blood pressure devices, and labs, and by get-ting almost all of the large retailers in this country—Wal-Mart, Kmart, Al-bertsons, CVS, Longs—to take mercury fever thermometers off their shelves. It has also worked to get hospitals to end the use of chlorine bleach.

We've worked a lot on the problems of polyvinyl chloride (PVC) plas-tic, the predominant plastic used in health care. All of us know PVC—it's in our new plastic shower curtain and our vinyl car seats. PVC is hard by na-ture, and to make it soft and clear enough to mold into medical tubing, you have to add phthalates. Tubing can be up to 80 percent phthalates by weight. It contains more phthalates than it does PVC. What happens over time, or if the PVC is exposed to too much heat, is that the phthalates can come out of the PVC and leak into the contents, into the medicine that's going through the tube, or the medicine that's in the IV bag. It's the same thing that occurs when old vinyl cracks. The phthalates have come out of the vinyl and gotten into the air, or into the product. Phthalates are a big health problem, especially for the developing male.

We've worked very hard to get the FDA to recognize that we can do better than using plastics that need to have phthalates in them for health care uses. More important, we've worked to get the world of health care to take responsibility for both the volume and the toxicity of waste it produces and to make widely known the successful alternatives—from hospitals that give away their kitchen waste for composting to organic farms that then sell produce to the hospitals, to places that have figured out how to recycle almost everything, to health care systems that have demanded and won reduced packaging or just made overall smart reduce-recycle-reuse decisions.

The health care sector in this country can be up to 30 percent of the gross national product, depending on how you calculate it. Anything we can do in health care to shift toward greener and buildings and cleaner materials will have a major impact. We must learn to no longer think that the way to solve problems is to shift the risk among patients, workers, and the environment, and instead actually figure out clever ways to reduce the risk and adopt a weight-of-the-evidence, burden-of-proof, precautionary approach. If we can figure out how to solve the problems in health care, that experience will give us the capacity to solve other problems that now seem insurmountable.

In all of the victories that we've won—and it's really been surprising what we've been able to win since 1996—the leadership of female nurses and other women health care workers has been paramount. The overwhelming majority of the doubters and the naysayers in industry have been male. Twenty years ago Carol Gilligan wrote *In a Different Voice*, an extraordinary work about women's psychological development and the difference between moral decision making among women and that among men. In it she quotes Sigmund Freud, who says, "Women show less sense of justice than men, that they are less ready to submit to the great demands of life, that they are more often influenced in their judgments by feelings of affection or hostility."

Gilligan also mentions Jean Piaget, who did the seminal studies of children's mental development. Piaget noted that as children grow up, the play of boys becomes increasingly focused on the legal elaboration of rules and the development of procedures to resolve conflicts. Girls, he observed, do not share this fascination. For girls, rules are pragmatic. Rules only matter if they make the game better. As soon as they don't, girls are ready to make exceptions. "This tendency," says Gilligan, "towards pragmatic tolerance led Piaget to conclude that the legal sense which is essential to moral development is far less developed in girls than in boys."

For Freud, for Piaget, and for all the psychologists and psychiatrists and child development specialists that followed and all the curriculums we grew up with, to grow into full moral beings, women, and men who might find themselves thinking like women, had to disconnect themselves from relationships, from responsibilities, from love, from caring, and become autonomous. Health for them wasn't membership; it was separateness.

Psychologists, including Lawrence Coleberg and Robert Kramer, describe six stages of moral development from childhood to adulthood. On level three, morality is seen in interpersonal terms. Level-three morality is helping others. Beginning at stage four, rules become more important than relationships. At the fifth and sixth, the "highest" stages, relationships become subordinate to universal principles.

Girls' morality, the "lesser" kind, is about relationships and responsibilities. Male morality, the "higher" kind, is about rights and rules. Objectivity is the highest moral value. Making things better is for moral weaklings.

So how does that definition of higher and lower morality translate to health care? If objectivity is the highest moral value, we build medicine as a scientific field of replicable proofs of cause and effect: Tuberculosis is caused by a bacillus, athlete's foot comes from a fungus, older mothers have a higher rate of Down's syndrome children. Of course, proving cause and effect is good, but when you try to figure out how people get sick, when you try to figure out the link between health and the environment, proving cause and effect can be almost impossible because of the innate complexity of these interactions.

We may never have absolute legal proof that a particular child's learning or behavior problems come from mercury exposure, or that dioxin from a certain incinerator causes endometriosis or other health problems, or that an increase in birth defects of the penis and human male infertility are conclusively caused by phthalates. So the current medical and legal model is stuck with a set of rules that don't fit reality. The rules tell us to look for a single cause of disease. The rules make medicine focus on clinically proven treatment rather than on logical but unproven methods of prevention. Medicine favors objective surgery over the subjective alleviation of suffering. We can't prove that taking action to reduce dioxin, to phase out PVC, to stop using mercury, or to reduce air pollution will reduce a particular patient's disease. It isn't like an appendectomy, a proven cure for a particular patient with a unique set of symptoms.

In medicine, what we can't prove, we ignore. In a world where the health of industry matters more than the planet and life upon it, industry keeps raising the bar for how much proof you need before you can take action. Fortunately, in nursing, we're held to a lower standard. We are forbidden to diagnose. That logical ordering of facts to reach a conclusion is too objective for our training. We are not a moral level-six profession. We are licensed level threes. We are there to help. As "lower" moral beings, nurses are allowed to think that information can be put to good use, even if it doesn't add up to absolute proof. Observations matter. Emotions matter. Intuition matters. Warnings can be listened to if there's something logical and practical you can do to stop the problem before it gets any bigger. We are naïve enough to think that it is more important, more moral to do something to help than it is to win a rule-laden game.

In Health Care without Harm, this thinking like a girl, in nurses and in non-nurses, in women and in men willing to think like girls, has allowed us to win many significant victories. Not in Congress, not in the courts, not in the arenas where the rules are everything, but in hospitals, clinics, markets, and communities around the world. Some fish have less mercury, breast milk has less dioxin, and baby boys will soon have less phthalate exposure because we're giving people permission and practical ways to think like girls.

I want to suggest to all of you that thinking like a girl is good medicine for each of us and for the world we live in. It's important to recognize that it wasn't the gods but a bunch of guys who decided that rules matter more than relationships and that the highest values should be based on objectivity and the subjugation of feelings. It wasn't God's own truth; it was their opinion. And opinions can be changed.

Redesigning
Environmental Health

Anthony Cortese

Dr. Anthony Cortese is one of the elders of ecological medicine. He was writing and speaking about it before it had a name.

Tony has made original contributions to the field of environmental education and long sought to build a bridge between environmental awareness and medicine. As president of Second Nature, he directed a visionary initiative to make environmental sustainability foundational to all higher education. He was the founder and managing director of the Consortium for Environmental Education in Medicine and served as the first dean of environmental programs at Tufts University. He founded both the Center for Environmental Management and the Tufts Environmental Literacy Institute, which received a presidential award from President George H. W. Bush in 1990.

As a public servant, he acted as commissioner of the Massachusetts Department of Environmental Protection and as an official at the EPA and the U.S. Public Health Service. He serves on many boards of directors and advisory committees. He is also a founding member and current chairman of the Natural Step U.S. and has been a consultant to the United Nations Environment Programme (UNEP). He is also an elected fellow of the American Association for the Advancement of Science (AAAS).

Tony's long and distinguished career in environmental activism and public service has made him a giant in the field of environmental education and policy. He continues to be at the cutting edge of the ecological literacy movement at all scholastic levels.

❀   ❀   ❀

PHYSICIANS DO GET TRAINED in the relationship of environment to health at most medical schools. That's the good news. The bad news is it's six hours in four years of medicine, which represents a 50 percent increase in the last fifteen years. The World Health Organization defines health as "a state of complete physical, mental and social well being, and not merely the absence of disease or infirmity." That definition leaves out any relationship to the natural world. It's based on the assumption that we are separate from nature. Why is it that we allow potentially toxic chemicals to be considered innocent until proven guilty? It has nothing to do with science. It's really the result of an assumption that whatever humans do to the environment is automatically, by definition, an improvement, because we are the pinnacle of creation, the dominant species, and we are separate from the rest of nature.

The state of one's environment is one of the most important determinants of health. Indeed, a healthy environment is one of the most important and fundamental factors in illness prevention and health promotion, and yet it is barely recognized by medicine. Communicating the idea that ecological health equals human health is absolutely critical. And the environmental health concerns we have today are no longer related just to pollution and waste but include exposure to altered environments and novel disease agents resulting from our encroaching on and exceeding the carrying capacity of natural systems. The alteration and disruption of biogeochemical cycles in ecosystems may be the most harmful thing we have ever done to ourselves.

Why don't physicians understand this? Global ecosystems provide services that humans cannot do without: food, fiber, fuel, shelter, water, a breathable atmosphere (thanks to photosynthesis), soil formation and fertility, climate regulation, pollination, natural pest control, the cycling of nutrients, the maintenance of biological diversity, the mitigation of floods and coastal erosion, and mental well-being, to mention only a few. An example important to me is the extraction of pharmaceutical drugs from nature. At least 25 percent of all the pharmaceutical drugs available today are derived from plants. I had acute leukemia over twenty-three years ago. At the time I was commissioner of the Department of Environmental Protection. It was ironic that I was trying to protect public health and the environment and I came down with acute leukemia. The chance that I would survive more than two years was about 10—20 percent. But one of the reasons I'm alive is because of a then experimental drug derived from the rosy periwinkle in the forests of Madagascar, 90 percent of which have been cut down. How many other lifesaving drugs are we destroying as a result of destroying ecosystems?

All these services provided by the natural world are free. Some ecological economists have estimated that if you were to value them from an economic standpoint, they would represent somewhere between $20 and $60 trillion per year. The mean estimate was $33 trillion a year. What that means is simply that if we didn't have these free services courtesy of the natural world, we'd have to spend another $33 trillion to get the $20 trillion economy that we have today, if money and technology could provide these services. These services cannot be replaced at any price: You can't substitute air for water, water for food, food for warmth and shelter, energy for air, technology for photosynthesis.

Ecological medicine is radically different from a bioengineering model of medicine in that it considers whether the relationship between humans and the natural world is in sync or not. It says we should be practicing medicine that works with nature and not against it, and it requires that all people who are practicing medicine understand evolution and ecological principles.

For example, if you look at the causes of current health problems, many of them are the result of food, chemicals, or environments to which we have not had the time and ability to evolve and adapt, such as fatty acids. Why, besides lack of physical activity, are so many people obese? We have an evolutionarily based craving for fat. Thirty-five thousand years ago we ate meat once a month, and those who could store fat could survive the longest. Now we eat large amounts of fatty acids daily and our health is suffering severely. Understanding how the environment has changed is crucial to analyzing and addressing many illnesses.

At the beginning of the 1900s, the average life span was about forty years in the developed world. It's now close to eighty years. But only seven years of that forty-year increase are attributable to modern medicine, according to Dr. Dick Jackson, director of the Center for Environmental Health at the Centers for Disease Control. Ninety percent of the reduction in the death rate occurred before the introduction of antibiotics or vaccines. It was largely due to improved water, food, and milk sanitation; a reduction in physical crowding; the introduction of central heating, municipal sewer systems, and refrigeration; and the move away from highly toxic coal and wood burning to less toxic natural gas and oil. Again, a change in the environment.

Virtually every woman who gets pregnant has morning sickness or nausea in the first trimester of pregnancy. A biologist name Marge Profet reasoned that something nearly everybody experiences must have a useful evolutionary purpose. She started doing research and found that the fetus is most vulnerable to toxins in the first trimester of pregnancy. After that, its vulnerability drops off by a factor of ten to twenty. So women's bodies are telling them that eating bland foods and foods with lower risks of toxicity (lower on the food chain, free of pesticides, and so forth) seems like a really important thing to do in the first trimester. Interestingly, studies also indicate that when a doctor gives a woman anti-nausea medication, or she just doesn't have nausea during the first trimester of pregnancy, there is actually a higher risk of birth defects and miscarriage. Again, this insight reaffirms that if we don't understand the evolutionary basis of our bodies' responses and their ecological context, we can't practice medicine in the right way, and in fact, we can actually do more harm than good. And what did Hippocrates tell us? First, do no harm.

Contemporary chronic diseases such as cancer, heart disease, diabetes, obesity, asthma, and depression are all diseases whose rates can be moderated by how we design and build our communities. In fact, land-use planning and zoning have their roots in a desire to protect the public's health. Again, Dr. Dick Jackson tells us that as far back as 1926, the U.S. Supreme Court argued that public health protection was one of the most basic responsibilities of local government, thus giving local government a legal mandate to restrict or control land-use decisions in a given community. Land-use decisions directly affect health. Sprawl is major cause of health problems. Since 1960, the amount of driving—per capita vehicle miles of travel—has increased by 250 percent. We add 90,000 new automobiles to the roads every day. We turn 364 acres of farmland or forest into developed land every hour in the United States.

Consider the health impacts. People walk less and less, and we have an epidemic of obesity. Sixty-one percent of the adult population in the United States is either overweight or obese as defined by the World Health Organization and the surgeon general. The number of obese children has more than doubled in the last twenty years. Asthma rates among children in the United States have more than doubled in the last fifteen years. During the 1996 Olympic Games in Atlanta, the city restricted driving and reduced traffic by about 22 or 23 percent. Smog was reduced by roughly 30 percent, and emergency visits to the hospital for asthma went down by 42 percent.

We find ourselves in a situation in which half the elderly and the disabled live within two blocks of a bus stop, but many of them cannot get to the bus stop because there are no sidewalks. We have designed the transportation systems in our communities around automobiles, not around people. Studies show that people who want to be more physically active are far more likely to be if they have access to nice scenery and a natural environment, and if it is safe. People will not go out and exercise if it is not safe. That's also an important public health problem, and we ought to be paying attention to it as such. Further, we need to consider the impact of sprawl on water quality. Every time you pave over an acre of prairie, that acre creates sixteen times as much polluted runoff as it did before. By paving too much land, we create contamination and disturb the hydrological cycle.

We have to have a different model for the practice of medicine. The people who practice medicine have to team up with architects, planners, and the engineers who are designing buildings and transportation systems, and start thinking about how we can provide access to as many people as possible, how we can create communities where people don't have to get into their cars to go to work, and where children can play without fear that they're going to be run over by a car. Of the automobile fatalities that occur in the United States, 13 percent are pedestrian fatalities, and 60 percent of those could be eliminated if we had redesigned the roads and there were actually sidewalks and cross-walks for people. Right now we don't think about human health when we design most communities.

As Dr. Howard Frumkin, professor at Emory Medical School, said, "If someone blew up a hospital or infected a water supply, we'd view it as an act of health terrorism. But pumping persistent organic pollutants into the at-mosphere, clearing forests, over-using resources and contributing to global warming are equally inimical to health." We are concerned now about the im-pact of terrorism on our health and survival. International security is absolutely necessary for protecting public health. The reverse is also true. If we provided sanitation to the 2.7 billion people without it, clean drinking water to the 1.1 billion people without it, food for the billion people who are malnourished, and decent housing for everyone, the seeds of terrorism would not be likely to take root. In the same way, if we want to change behavior to protect the en-vironment, we need to emphasize the public health angle, because most people will change their behavior only if they see it's in their self-interest. So it's po-litically intelligent to connect what we're trying to do to protect the environ-ment with its impact on our health and well-being. The more coalitions we can bring together, the greater the change we can make in public policy and the better our chances of success in making ecological medicine the wave of the future.

Generations at Risk:
Children's Health and the Environment

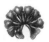

Ted Schettler

Dr. Ted Schettler's penetrating gray eyes convey a paradoxical mix of play and gravitas. Perhaps it's because his special interest—the effects of environmental toxins on children's health and development—gives him an especially poignant window onto a world where the health of the young of many species is jeopardized by the unwise use of industrial chemicals and shortsighted ecosystem destruction.

Ted serves on the staff of Boston Medical Center and has a clinical practice at the East Boston Neighborhood Health Center. He has also worked extensively with community groups and nongovernmental organizations (NGOs) addressing the health effects of environmental contamination and toxic exposures. He is the coauthor of two seminal works on children's health and environmental pollutants, Generations at Risk: Reproductive Health and the Environment *and* In Harm's Way: Toxic Threats to Child Development. *He is the science director of the Science and Environmental Health Network and co-chair of the Human Health and Environment Project of Greater Boston Physicians for Social Responsibility. He serves on a variety of local, state, and national environmental health committees.*

He has tirelessly educated the medical profession and citizens' groups on the precautionary principle. In the case of children, Ted knows all too well that an ounce of prevention is worth more than fifty pounds of cure.

Ted's work could prove to be decisive for the success of the ecological medicine movement. Children are often at greatest risk from environmental factors, and harm to children entails profound costs for the individual, family, community, and ecosystem. The young of all species are the most vulnerable, and they are the future.

❦   ❦   ❦

I AM A PHYSICIAN with an additional degree in public health who has spent a lot of time studying environmental health issue. Over the past ten or more years I have been looking at the impacts of environmental contaminants and environmental factors on human health in general, but focusing especially on reproductive health and childhood development.

Health depends on a number of interactive factors—genetic, environmental, social, political, economic, and so on. For example, a person who is living in a socially deprived or marginal circumstance is often more susceptible for one reason or another to environmental impacts, and people who have certain genetic makeups may be more vulnerable in some ways to a specific environmental exposure. So we can't completely separate these factors, and we shouldn't try, but we need to try to understand them and how they affect each other. Many people in the medical mainstream don't quite seem to understand that these factors interact in complex ways.

Why are children more at risk from negative environmental factors? Developing tissues are often inherently more susceptible than those of adults, and children are frequently disproportionately exposed to environmental factors. Then, as Dr. Phil Landrigan of Mount Sinai School of Medicine in New York says, "Children have a longer shelf life than adults." They're going to be around longer. They have a longer time to experience the outcomes from early life events. A child grows from a single cell into a walking, talking, social, intelligent, interactive human being in two or three years. That's a remarkable story of growth and development: A whole lot has gone on during that time, and a lot can go wrong. Many of the body's systems are not yet fully developed, whether it's the brain, reproductive system, hormones, lungs, or liver.

Children double their weight in just three months. They absorb many contaminants and nutrients from their intestinal tract much more readily than adults. For example, a child has to absorb a lot of calcium from the intestine to build a skeleton. Children also absorb lead much more quickly and rapidly from the intestine than an adult does. So a smaller exposure that might not affect an adult can damage a child.

The first environment is the womb. We used to be taught in medical school that the placenta serves as a barrier to environmental contaminants that a mother may have been exposed to, but actually that's largely untrue. Almost anything a pregnant woman internalizes from the outside world that gets circulated in her blood can make it across the placenta. Some compounds do so much more quickly than others, but virtually everything can ultimately get across. Babies are basically exposed to what their mother is exposed to, although there may be some difference in the amounts.

We can measure lead, mercury, pesticides, and other toxins in a baby. A small study that looked at the first bowel movements of babies and analyzed them for organophosphate pesticides found that all had more than one organophosphate pesticide residue in their bowel movement, and most had five or six. We know with certainty that children are being exposed to organophosphate pesticides in utero. That's been clearly demonstrated.

Proportionate to their size, children take in far more air, food, and water than adults, so their exposures to toxins are higher. Also, children's eating habits often involve latching onto a particular food group and eating lots of it, so if there are pesticide residues on that specific type of food, they will be exposed at a higher rate than an adult eating a more varied diet. Furthermore, children spend far more time on the floor or near the floor than adults do. They crawl around on carpets and then stick their hands in their mouths. Carpets are a tremendous repository for pesticides. Carpets actually turn out to be the largest source of pesticide exposure for most children. The dust that accumulates in indoor environments is contaminated with pesticides. It's estimated that about 70 percent of a child's total pesticide exposure comes from indoor dust.

Children breathe closer to the ground, of course, and some chemicals tend to accumulate lower in a room because they're heavier than air. Pound for pound, children breathe more than adults do when they go outside and play. They're often more active than adults and they're exposed to bigger doses of outdoor air contaminants such as ozone and particulates.

Studies have shown a direct correlation between children's exposure to air pollutants and their likelihood of having an asthma attack. But new information goes a step further, showing that air pollutants can actually cause asthma—not just trigger an asthma attack in a person who has the condition, but actually cause it. Some of the research was done in Southern California and measured ozone exposure.

Advocates of chemicals and their widespread use argue that the dose makes the poison, that large amounts of anything can hurt you, and that because our exposures are very low, we don't need to worry. But any good toxicology textbook will tell you that the timing, pattern, and duration of an exposure to a toxin can be as important as dosage. Even small exposures in a developing child that occur during certain windows of vulnerability can have an impact that may be long lasting or permanent, whereas if that same exposure had happened days, weeks, or months later, it would have had little or no impact. We have seen in animal brain studies that an exposure on a certain day during embryonic development may have one set of impacts, and that the same exposure three days later can produce a totally different set of impacts.

The age-adjusted incidence of some cancers continues to increase. These include skin cancers such as melanoma, breast and lung cancers in women, kidney cancer, bladder cancer, lymphoma, prostate cancer, testicular cancer, and others. These illnesses have multiple causes, but we've suspected for some time that early life exposures in children can increase the risk of developing certain childhood cancers. We now have evidence to suggest that early life exposures can actually have an impact that manifests itself much later, anywhere along the timeline of our aging. A widely known case is that of women who were administered DES during pregnancy back in the 1950s and 1960s. Their daughters had a much higher risk of a rare form of vaginal cancer that showed up twenty or thirty years later. There's now increasing evidence to suggest that a number of cancers may actually be the result of very early life exposures.

Two important papers were published in the *International Journal of Cancer* in the summer of 2002. They involved the study of a Swedish database that looked at the detailed medical histories of 9.6 million people—not a small study. The bottom line was that for *all* cancers, even those known to have a high genetic component, environmental factors were more important than genetics. The second key finding was that cancer risk is largely established during the first twenty years of life. People who migrate from one country to another before they're twenty years old tend to acquire the cancer risk of the country that they move to. If they immigrate after they're twenty years old, they tend to keep the cancer risk of the country that they came from. Asian women living in Asia have a much lower risk of breast cancer than Caucasian women living in the United States, but Asian women who are born in the United States or who move here young have nearly the same cancer risk as Caucasian women in the same environment. It's the early years that seem to matter most.

We are also becoming increasingly aware that, in addition to obvious structural birth defects, we need to pay attention to functional birth defects. We know lead exposure in the womb impairs brain development, for example. You won't see that looking at the child's body, but it may become apparent that the child's cognitive abilities are not developing normally. We should get in the habit of calling that a birth defect. It's the result of an in-utero exposure that leads to a significant and measurable health problem and has functional impacts down the road.

We're seeing now that even low exposures to chemicals that can mimic hormones in the womb can sometimes reprogram certain systems in the body, such as the nervous, neuroendocrine, and reproductive systems, so that they can't function properly later in life. We are accumulating more and more human data indicating that environmental contaminants such as certain solvents and pesticides are implicated in increasing the risk of birth defects. For example, a study done in Minnesota showed that pesticide applicators were far more likely than the norm to father children with birth defects, and the birth defect risk was higher if a child was conceived in the spring, which is the time of highest pesticide use.

Learning disabilities, attention-deficit/hyperactivity disorder (ADHD), and perhaps autism seem to be on the rise. It's hard to be absolutely certain there has been a real increase in autism, rather than just improved reporting or improved record keeping, but there's been a 210 percent increase in cases reported to the California Autism Registry in the past thirteen years. A recent analysis of that database concluded that the increase in cases is not just the result of changed reporting requirements. The evidence suggests we are indeed seeing a real increase.

Why is a developing child's brain so vulnerable? Cells in the embryonic brain have to divide and then migrate to the place they belong in the brain. They don't start out where they belong. They must migrate along pathways that are established in the brain and then differentiate into various specialized cell types. They form connections known as synapses with their neighbors in order to set up complex neural networks, and then a lot of "pruning" of those synapses goes on for the first couple of years of life. That whole cascade of events needs to occur in a sequence, in an orderly fashion, for the result to come out right.

Many environmental contaminants such as lead, mercury, PCBs, pesticides, alcohol, tobacco smoke, and radiation can affect that cascade of events at one place or another, or at several places. We now know that lead, for example, can impair IQ, learning, and attention and is associated with hyperactivity and impulsive-aggressive behavior. This, by the way, has economic and social impacts as well as purely medical costs. Who is bearing the cost? It's the individual affected, of course, but also the family and the whole community.

Mercury is another highly dangerous toxin. Most of us are exposed to mercury through a variety of sources, including air and water pollution, contaminated fish we eat, and, for some, mercury dental fillings. Mercury easily crosses the placenta and gets into the developing fetal brain, where it can be very disruptive. High levels are associated with mental retardation, cerebral palsy, problems walking, delayed psychomotor development, and seizures. That's been observed among populations in locales where there have been accidental poisoning episodes. But far lower levels of exposure in utero and in early childhood are associated with impaired memory and learning and atten-tion problems later in life. Those exact traits are what we see popping up in the diagnosing of ADHD.

With ADHD there's no question that there's also a genetic component, but that is not the whole story. A child exposed to lead or mercury in the womb will have problems with attention, impulsiveness, and learning. We need to spread the word about all these findings because when you start talking about real threats to kids' brain development, people start paying attention, as they should. We have compelling opportunities to take the solid, convincing sci-entific research that has accumulated in this field and use it in campaigns to alert people and communities that those they cherish and love most, their chil-dren, are at risk, but that the risks are preventable, if we heed the science and take action.

Part II

The "Duh" Principle: Precaution Means Not Having to Say You're Sorry

The Precautionary Principle:
Golden Rule for the New Millennium

Carolyn Raffensperger

Carolyn Raffensperger has helped define, shape, and lead the ecological medicine move-ment. She and her team at the nonprofit Science and Environmental Health Network have purposefully sown the seeds of its centerpiece, the precautionary principle, across the United States.

She is among the preeminent precautionary visionaries. She has one of those dazzling free-ranging minds that's constantly making offbeat connections. She does it with enormous grace and kindness, with the careful ear of a trained listener, and with the fairness of a citizen diplomat bridging many worlds. In her heart she carries the fiery commitment of an ardent defender of the rights of all life, both human and nonhuman.

Carolyn has a varied background reflective of her far-reaching interests. She's the proud daughter of a Chicago surgeon who himself became a passionate environmentalist after noticing patterns linking cancers and birth defects in children to environmental factors. An anthropologist by training, she studied the ancient Anasazi culture in the Four Corners area of the Southwest. She went on to law school and worked with the Sierra Club for nine years. She served on committees for the National Research Council and the EPA on numerous topics, from risk assessment to pesticides to radioactive waste.

In 1995, she became executive director of the Science and Environmental Health Network, a singularly important think tank and information clearinghouse dedicated to public-interest science and to democratizing science for the common good. She coedited the seminal book Protecting Public Health and the Environment: Implementing the Precautionary Principle. *She has also been a farmer in North Dakota, where she and her Biodynamic farmer husband, Fred Kirschenmann, grew much of their own food. She has spoken everywhere from Harvard and the White House to meetings of chemical manufacturers and of small towns defending their local environments. Most recently, she has taken on the legal profession, organizing workshops around the country on how industry is increasingly feeding junk science to the courts in order to dumb down environmental protection.*

❀　　❀　　❀

LIKE MANY OF YOU, I've been mesmerized and horrified by the events that have transpired since the morning of September 11, 2001. During this difficult time I've been trying to compose my thoughts and write. What could I possibly say within the context of terrorism and war that would have any meaning?

Well, it turns out that Donald Rumsfeld, President Bush, John Ashcroft, and the Florida Department of Health have all had something to say on the topic of precaution. According to the leaders of the U.S. government, they are taking every precaution to protect the citizens of the United States.

But I am not sure they get it. Consider this: One day last week we were told that the only goal of the war on terrorism is to protect Americans. Only minutes later we were told that it is 100 percent certain that there will be further acts of terrorism against Americans because of our retaliatory actions. If preventing harm to Americans is the goal, then why are we doing something that guarantees harm with 100 percent certainty?

This reminds me of a quote by the great author Joseph Conrad, who said, "Let them think what they like, but I didn't mean to drown myself. I meant to swim until I sank—but that's not the same thing."

Perhaps the environmental lessons we've learned about the precautionary principle might be helpful to Rumsfeld et al. Let me share some of those lessons with you in their absence.

We've transformed our world in a very short period of time—at least from the vantage point of other living things. Technology dominates all aspects of our lives. From medicine to agriculture, energy, communication, and transportation, we have technologies our grandparents could not have imagined and that now shadow our world.

What is striking is that we have not had a parallel transformation of ideas. Science, government, and law are mummified in ideas developed hundreds of years ago. Bacon and Descartes, Locke and Smith are still the key thinkers we use to decide about technologies. Our ideas have not changed so that they guide us to truth and justice—much less beauty and health—in the face of our destructive capacities.

I doubt that we humans mean to drown ourselves in our waste or foolishness—in the dark side of our technologies. I suspect we think we'll just swim until we sink amid global warming, endocrine disruption, the loss of biodiversity, and our capacities for destruction through war and terrorism.

There is another choice beyond drowning and sinking. This third choice, this life raft, requires hard work, humility, respect. It embodies that which is good and right and that which is beautiful. Some have called this third choice the precautionary principle. I would submit to you that the precautionary principle is one of a handful of ideas with truly transformative power.

I would like to do two things here: First, describe the precautionary principle and a process for implementing it; second, lay out how science, agriculture, medicine, and law can be transformed by the precautionary principle.

The concept of the precautionary principle comes from Germany. The words "precautionary principle" were translated from the German *Vorsorgeprinzip*. A more literal translation of *Vorsorge* is "forecaring"—to care into the future. The Germans use *Vorsorge* in the sense of preparing for what may be a difficult future.

For thirty years the precautionary principle has been used widely in Europe, mostly with regard to toxic chemicals. But in the United States it is best known as a provision in the preamble of the 1992 environmental treaty known as the Rio Declaration. The Rio Declaration says this: "Where there are threats of serious or irreversible damage, lack of full scientific certainty shall not be used as a reason for postponing cost-effective measures to prevent environmental degradation."

While not poetic, the Rio Declaration contains the core precautionary principle elements: scientific uncertainty, the likelihood of harm, and precautionary action.

Up until 1998, the precautionary principle was a rather nebulous, ethereal idea. It was stuck in treaty preambles or viewed as a baseless belief. In 1998, we convened the Wingspread conference to get it unstuck and put it into motion.

The Wingspread definition of the precautionary principle is as follows: "When an activity raises threats of harm to human health or the environment, precautionary measures should be taken even if some cause and effect relationships are not fully established scientifically." The Wingspread statement went on to lay out four elements of implementing the principle.

First, people have a duty to take anticipatory action to prevent harm. (This is really a restatement of the precautionary principle.) Second, the burden of proof for a new technology, process, activity, or chemical lies with the proponents, not with the public. Another way to frame this is that the polluter must pay for damage.

The notion that the burden of proof rests with the proponents announces up front that society will hold someone accountable. It provides a real impetus for proponents to think carefully about proposed activities before they undertake something hazardous. Is this activity necessary? Are there other ways to accomplish the same ends? And if prevention fails, there is a backup plan. The public isn't forced to absorb the costs of the damage.

Of course, we are all culpable and we are all responsible for damaging activities. At the same time, there are some technologies or activities where the proponent has more information—or should have more information— about potential harms as well as uncertainties, and so has a greater obligation to prevent damage.

The third mechanism for implementing the precautionary principle is that people have an obligation to examine "a full range of alternatives" before starting a new activity, whether it is using a new chemical or a new technology. If this activity is potentially harmful, do we have other options that are less destructive? For instance, if we were to get serious about ending starvation, are there alternatives to biotechnology? Or is that the only method to feed the hungry?

Fourth, decisions applying the precautionary principle must be "open, informed, and democratic" and "must include affected parties." The reason that the precautionary principle requires democratic participation is that when we make decisions that are unresolvable with science, they are, by their very nature, ethical and political. And too, by involving affected parties we are more likely to get far better science and a better array of options.

Since Wingspread we've identified other steps for implementing the precautionary principle. One is to set a goal or establish a vision—to know where you are trying to go. For instance, the Swedish people decided that their goal was that no child would be born with toxic chemicals in its body. The goal itself is precautionary. But the mechanisms for achieving the goal must also comply with precaution.

Perhaps the biggest surprise since Wingspread has been uncovering and discovering the deep ethical dimensions of the precautionary principle. As environmentalists, we knew well the ideas of scientific uncertainty and harm. Many of us got so we could discuss the ins and outs of type I and type II errors, indeterminacy, and the relative merits and problems of reductionism. Many of us are motivated to use the precautionary principle because we see damage in the world, whether it is the cancer of a loved on, the loss of a critter, or the sense that the world is heating up. But ethics? Values? No way. We just didn't know how to talk about them.

But here lies the power of the precautionary principle. It tells us to make decisions with both heart and mind. Too often, we have been told that emotions, values, things we love are irrelevant. We've been told that Science is King. But King Science is held captive by narrow economic interests. Other values have been cast aside. We have sacrificed the environment and public health on the altar of economic gain.

In 2000, a group met at Blue Mountain to explore the values that are the foundation of the precautionary principle. That group decided something interesting. They came to the conclusion that values or ethics aren't just nice things we need to get along with each other but that they are essential for survival.

Here are some of the values: "Our life depends on *gratitude*. Our life depends on *empathy*, because we are connected with all of creation. Our life depends on *compassion, humility, respect, simplicity*." And perhaps my favorite: "Our life depends on *humor*, because life is good, and humor disrobes tyranny and absurdity." The Blue Mountain statement ends with this lovely sentence: "It is through love for the particular—a child, a neighborhood, a family of otters, a meandering river—that we find our way to a sustaining relationship with the Earth and our communities."

Is the precautionary principle enough to bring about a transformation of environmental policy? I think so.

The old idea of waiting until we can count the dead bodies has failed. We keep thinking we can do risk assessments on things for which we cannot even imagine worst-case scenarios. How do we do risk assessments on Yucca Mountain, which must contain radioactive waste for 10,000 years? How do we do a risk assessment on an ocean that drives our climate and is soon going to be warmer than our bathtub? How do we do a risk assessment on an entire generation of children who can only cope by being drugged with Ritalin or Prozac?

This is why I believe the precautionary principle is the beginning of an essential transformation in the way we relate both to the earth and to the things we invent. The chorus that we should hear, what we should listen to, is the voice of our children, which we should obey and heed. We can set a goal for a beautiful, livable, healthy world. But in order to meet that goal we will have to transform some of the pillars of our society: science, agriculture, medicine, and law.

Let me describe the necessary transformations, beginning with science.

As I described earlier, scientific uncertainty is key to the precautionary principle. The uncertainty is usually about cause and effect—did this chemical or will this chemical damage children's brains, frogs' legs, or the ozone layer? Will logging reduce the habitat of Julia Butterfly Hill and grizzly bears? Is fossil fuel consumption really causing global climate change?

What opponents of environmental protection would have us believe is that we should wait for the old eighteenth-century science to provide conclusive answers before we take precautionary actions. This is a recipe for big trouble: Wait until the dead bodies of trees, children, and salmon are piled in the streets before we take action.

Fortunately, we don't have to wait. We can take science back and have it serve the public good rather than corporate profits. The former president of the American Association for the Advancement of Science, Jane Lubchenco, has called for a new social contract for science. She graciously acknowledges that the old contract scientists had with the public has been fulfilled. Science provided cures for infectious disease so our life expectancy has gone up. And science provided for national security with the Manhattan Project. But the contract must now change. She says that on this human-dominated planet we need to ask science to do something different—to help get us out of the environmental mess. All of life depends on the life support system of the earth. Science can help us understand that system and help restore the environment so it can continue to sustain life.

How should we go about doing that, especially since we don't understand complex biological systems? When we don't know how a chemical is going to function or what the consequences of an activity might be, we have to live by some basic biological principles even when we are missing specific facts. The Natural Step, for instance, lays out ecological systems conditions that are precautionary, and these I think are absolute floors, not ceilings. These are the bare minimum that is going to let us survive. They say society should not produce substances faster than they can be broken down by natural processes. Nor should society extract resources at a faster rate than they're replenished, for example, by overharvesting trees or fish. I call this one the "duh" factor. Maybe actually we should call the precautionary principle the "duh" principle.

Then we need to at least follow these bare minimum system conditions and design technologies that are in concert with living systems, not just in concert with economic systems. Some wonderful scientists are pointing the direction. Terry Collins, the genius chemist, is laying the foundation of green chemistry. He begins by saying how nature works. Nature uses few chemicals to do lots of things. In contrast, humans use many, many chemicals that are a threat to life, particularly the chlorinated compounds and heavy metals. Janine Benyus is another person doing precautionary science. She too is asking how the world works and then how we can mimic those processes.

I've laid out part of the scientists' end of the new social contract. But what about the public's part? If we really want green chemistry and green biology, green economics and green sociology, what do we need to do?

First, we should create a public-interest precautionary research agenda. We've allowed special interests—primarily corporations—to dominate the research agenda and to use publicly funded research to make more profits. Corporations like Monsanto have enough money; they don't need the public's money as well. We must tell our legislators what a public-interest research agenda would look like. And then we need to fund it.

Second, graduate school is the perfect time and place for young scientists to participate in public-interest research. What if we made graduate school more like the Peace Corps? It's a wonderful time for graduate students to dedicate a piece of research to the common good.

Third, we have to set up regulatory systems that treat every product or practice that is approved for the market as an experiment. That is, we have to monitor Bt corn, household cleaners, and logging and grazing regimes. Then we need to yank technologies and stop activities that we didn't accurately predict would be damaging. We simply cannot put profits over public health and the environment.

Now that is a tall order for science. But the impacts on our world—particularly agriculture and medicine—could be profound. Agriculture and medicine are both human attempts to come to terms with complex biological systems. The precautionary principle is crucial at this interface.

Agriculture is one of humanity's most destructive practices. Isn't it ironic that what should be an earthy, biological, nourishing process is in fact one of the most damaging and poisonous? As I was writing this, I began with a list of just what we've done to water in the name of agriculture. The list was so long I could have written a whole speech around the dead zone in the Gulf of Mexico, pfisteria, and soil erosion. I didn't even begin the energy, biodi-versity, or air pollution lists. If we can't apply the precautionary principle to agriculture and find a way to feed ourselves without destroying the planet, then the principle is worthless. It also means we are probably not educable as a species.

It seemed so easy for a while—use the bounties of nature for our own ad-vantage. Plant better, more, and bigger crops. Use more efficient methods, more chemicals, and technological advances ad infinitum. The precautionary prin-ciple is a direct challenge to that kind of singlemindedness, that kind of hubris. If we are to continue feeding ourselves, we have to step back and realize how big the unknowns have been and what the price has been of ignoring them. The principle is absolutely foreign to the cut-it-down, use-it-up, pour-on-the-chemicals, globalize, industrialize, tweak-the-technology approach of Amer-ican agriculture.

The precautionary principle calls for an end to such reckless behavior in the face of ignorance.

Where should we begin? As Fred Kirschenmann said in an article on agri-culture and the precautionary principle, "We've been asking what we can get away with rather than how to fit our farming into nature." Simply put, under the precautionary principle we will fit agriculture into nature rather than forc-ing nature to do our will. Here's the good news. There's a whole movement of people in sustainable agriculture who have pioneered the ecological pre-cautionary food system.

Medicine, like agriculture, is a profoundly biological activity that has con-tributed to the degradation of environmental health and at the same time is scrambling to treat the cancers, birth defects, reproductive disorders, and learn-ing disabilities caused by environmental degradation.

The precautionary principle calls for us to prevent environmental health damage even if we can't prove cause and effect. In one of its simplest mani-festations, the precautionary principle reflects the physicians' Hippocratic prin-ciple in its call to do no harm. And here we recognize that the precautionary principle is not so foreign to American medicine, even conventional medicine. We are careful about how we treat our bodies, what medicines we put into

them. Drugs are in principle submitted to the precautionary standard of doing no harm. And when they *do* harm, as many do, we are supposed to be told
what that is.

But this precautionary approach has been limited pretty much to what we
put into our bodies deliberately. It has not gone far enough. We have not taken
into account the fact that our bodies are not isolated from our surroundings,
that they are permeable and vulnerable. We have been careless about what
we expose our children to—we vaccinate them against all kinds of diseases
but subject them to all kinds of poisons in utero. And in a horrible twist, hospitals have been discharging mercury and dioxins into the environment and
then turning around and having to heal the very people made ill by their own
practices. This is crazy.

The precautionary principle calls for broader, more inclusive medical care-
taking. It calls for ecological medicine.

What, you might ask, is ecological medicine? Ecological medicine promotes environmental health. That is, it promotes the health of all species and
recognizes that their health—our health—is interdependent. The health of
the redwood, the health of the salmon, the health of the Afghani woman is
my health. And in the practice of promoting environmental health, ecological medicine doesn't cause more environmental damage. Isn't that a wonderful idea?

These activities of science, agriculture, and medicine all funnel back into
the law. The law is defined as the set of rules a community agrees to be bound
by. Unfortunately our law has been taken over by corporations, for corporations, leaving communities and precaution in their dust. Let me explain. Much
of our environmental work has focused on Congress and the EPA, not the
courts, because we assumed we could actually get justice through the judicial
system. But several separate but intertwined developments in the U.S. courts
have converged into a disturbing pattern: Increasingly, science is distorted in
ways that favor commercial and industrial interests and that work against the
broader public interest. The courts are still using that eighteenth-century science. To make matters worse, that old scientific system is being corrupted even
further by campaign financing and other antidemocratic political processes.

I believe that the lessons of the precautionary principle can promote justice in the courts, particularly where the science is uncertain. How so? We know that the precautionary principle requires democratic participation. And our legal system requires it, at least in theory—laws are supposedly established through a democratic process. But two aspects of our current judicial system are undemocratic and unprecautionary. First, corporate and industrial interests are able to buy the election of judges by paying for their campaigns. Campaign finance reform is necessary for Congress; it's even more important for the courts. More than forty states elect their judges. Some of the right-wing campaigns have spent millions of dollars for a single judgeship.

Second, increasingly, scientific evidence is being taken away from juries. Much of this is a result of a case known as *Daubert v. Merrell Dow Pharmaceuticals, Inc.* that the Supreme Court decided in 1993. This case strengthened the role of judges as gatekeepers for scientific evidence. Cases that followed encouraged judges to sift evidence and experts according to standards of "sound science" in order to prevent questionable scientific testimony from being presented to juries. Rather than placing responsibility for determining the validity of evidence and uncertainty with juries, this gave judges lots of room to act as experts themselves.

But this buzzword "sound science," invented by those who oppose environmental protection, has a limited meaning. It means you have to prove with certainty that my chemical caused your harm—exactly what the precautionary principle warns us will lead to more injury. Modern science has shown that some technologies or chemicals can damage future generations. We learned this the hard way from the drug DES, which did so much harm to the daughters of the women who took it. But the courts are not currently equipped to deal with the fact that some things cause damage in the future or far from the place they were used. So how does a terribly poisoned community in Louisiana or south Texas get justice? As it stands, the judicial system will extract blood but deny justice on the basis of this outdated science.

A wonderful legal scholar named Margaret Berger has suggested that having to prove that your chemical caused my injury is the wrong basis for liability. She says that the basis for liability should be simply whether a company has tested that chemical or not. This would be remarkable, because we know next to nothing about the more than 80,000 chemicals on the market.

There is one more idea I would like to add to this precautionary legal stew. The ideas used by the courts are really quite old—just like those of science. Many old things are worth keeping, but it helps to reexamine the context and to test the old ideas. The courts have been using a standard of law to decide almost everything but criminal cases. They have been using the reasonable person standard. Now, reasonableness is a good and valuable trait. It is quite useful even as a standard of law. But several years ago a colleague and I proposed a new standard of law for situations where reason doesn't quite fit—like offenses against dignity, and scientific uncertainty. This is the respectful person standard. When we have vast uncertainty and the harm could be great, it would be wise for us to be respectful. If we are, we will be far less likely to blunder our way into big trouble through ignorance and arrogance. The respectful person gives deference to the mysteries of this great and marvelous earth. This is inherently precautionary.

And so we are at a fork in the road. We can continue blundering into an impoverished, degraded, lonely earth devoid of other beings. The precautionary principle maps the possibility of the other choice—a good and whole and beautiful world.

There are many ways to kneel and kiss the earth.

Quantifying the Unknowable:
The Risks of Risk Assessment

Peter Montague

You would never know from Peter Montague's quiet humility and modesty that he has long been one of the environmental movement's authentic visionaries and one of the industrial juggernaut's most feared opponents.

He brings an unimpeachable expertise and penetrating intelligence to the gnarliest scientific and social issues without ever losing sight of the on-the-ground reality of human suffering so often masked by depersonalized studies. He has a mind-boggling capacity for digesting, analyzing, and explaining scientific data with impeccable clarity. He exhibits steadfast fairness in his quest to bring environmental health and justice into the world.

Peter is the cofounder and director of the Environmental Research Foundation (ERF), which is best known for Rachel's Environment and Health News, the superlative newsletter Peter edits and publishes. Named after Rachel Carson, the e-letter is consistently a source of the most urgently needed cutting-edge environmental health ideas and strategies. It's the closest thing to a crystal ball that environmental health advocates have.

But more than that, Peter's work provides grassroots pollution fighters with technical information in an understandable, useful form. In addition, he has helped connect environmental health activists across the country into potent networks whose whole is far greater than the sum of the parts. As an organizer, he is unparalleled.

Peter has coauthored two books on toxic heavy metals in the natural environment and has been ahead of the curve on countless environmental policy issues, from endocrine disrupters to the precautionary principle.

❀   ❀   ❀

THE WAY WE MAKE DECISIONS today started evolving around
1965, when the Cuyahoga River was catching on fire and other rivers were
bubbling with detergents. Things were obviously deteriorating pretty rapidly.
The federal government was writing reports about it. The White House was
concerned. It just didn't look good. A regulatory framework was developed.
And of course it was an intellectual apparatus that rested on assumptions.

This regulatory framework based on "risk assessment" is widely used today. It is used to site power plants—coal-burning or nuclear—or a medical
waste or garbage incinerator, or an industrial flaring operation to get rid of organic chemicals, or a new highway, or to decide how much of a pesticide is
safe to spray and how much is safe to leave on your food, or how big you can
make a garbage dump and still have it be a good neighbor.

It would be used to decide how clean to make a dump site where a lot of
dangerous material has been left by the military or by the private sector. The
logic is that you can't afford to clean up 100 percent, so you need to decide
how much you really need to clean up. Risk assessment will give you a precise numerical answer to that question, and thank God for those precise numerical answers! We all need them. Deciding how much traffic to allow in
a neighborhood, for example—how much air pollution can be tolerated in a
neighborhood—would be a risk assessment question. Setting limits on how
many fish you can sustainably catch in the ocean is a risk assessment question. Deciding how many trees you could take out of a certain section of a
national forest without destroying it as habitat for wildlife—that's a risk assessment question.

The philosophy of risk assessment is pervasive throughout the governments of the industrial world, with perhaps the exception of Germany and
some of the Scandinavian countries that are starting to move in a different direction. But the United States is hard-core risk assessment territory. We do
not use any other technique for making these decisions.

The first assumption of risk assessment is that we can know how much of an activity is dangerous or destructive. We can intellectually know that through scientific analysis, whether it's how much pesticide to spray or how many fish to take from the ocean without killing off all the fish.

The second assumption is that if there are dangers to this activity, we will learn of them before permanent or major damage has occurred. We are smart enough, discerning enough, clever enough, and observant enough to see the problems before they become overwhelmingly large and do us all in, or do in some other species, or cause permanent damage like harm the ozone layer of the planet, or create global warming. The risk assessment paradigm says that we will catch those things before they happen. It's obvious that the risk assessment paradigm doesn't work, but risk assessors still insist that this is a valid assumption.

The third assumption of the regulatory system is that we are smart enough to go chemical by chemical, activity by activity, factory by factory, river by river, ocean by ocean, everywhere in the United States, and by extension, everywhere on the planet, and set numerical limits to those activities so that the cumulative effect will not add up to an ecological disaster. That Herculean intellectual task is in fact the assumption of the risk assessment system, as astonishing as it may seem, and as arrogant as it may seem.

There's another assumption underlying this system, which is that the burden of proving harm is on the public. These activities are assumed to be beneficial, benign, and innocent until they are proven guilty. So any corporation can basically start up any new activity, or put some new chemical into the environment at will, and it is up to you and me to do the discerning, to gather the data, to put cause and effect together in a persuasive way, and to petition government to then put the clamps on this activity. If you've got an army of scientists and lawyers at your beck and call, you may have some chance, in a twenty-year litigated effort, of minimally reducing the harm that you have observed. With the presumption of innocence on the side of the polluters and the destroyers, you, the citizen who is simply trying to live your life and keep the planet functioning, have a very uphill battle in the current framework.

So what is a risk assessment? Risk assessment has been carefully codified by the federal government. You can buy a book on how to do a risk assessment; it's not an arbitrary exercise. It starts by deciding how toxic a chemical is and what exposures might occur and what damage those exposures might cause. It all sounds very rational, but when you really get into trying to decide how toxic a particular chemical is, you realize we don't even know what questions to ask about toxicity.

Ten years ago, nobody was asking "Do these chemicals interfere with our hormones?" They didn't even know that was a question to ask. There's real ignorance about what the damage might be. To figure out how dangerous a given chemical is is a giant intellectual task that basically cannot be done because we're so ignorant we don't even know what we're ignorant about. Because we don't know what we don't know, we often can't ask the right questions. We surely can never be so arrogant as to say that we know all the right questions to ask.

That first step of asking "How dangerous is this material?" is fraught with uncertainty. What we do is expose rats to a chemical, and then we say, "Well, rats really aren't like people." If we decide that sixty parts per million is safe for a rat based on some assessment of the rat's health, then we say, "People are really different from rats, and so let's protect people more than we protect rats, so we'll cut it by ten." Instead of sixty parts per million being safe for people, we'll say six parts per million is safe for people. Is that scientific? Why do we use ten? Because we have a numbering system based on ten? Why not use a factor of 11.65 or 200 or some other number? It's arbitrary, it's not scientific.

Then there's the question of exposure. Let's say a chemical is going to be released into the environment, say from an airplane, intended to hit only cotton plants. But there are always those uncooperative weather patterns and glitches in the system, and so without actually testing people's blood or urine or taking some other real measure of exposure, you make all kinds of assumptions. You start plugging in numbers to climate models: If the wind is from the west 45 percent of the time, and it's from the southwest 18 percent of the time, and if it's six miles an hour at night and eighteen miles an hour during the day, how much of X is going to impact community Z downwind?

I might as well just pull a number out of my ear as think that I'm going to be able to solve that really complicated set of factors and put them all into one equation and come out with one nice round number that is going to mean anything. I know it's hard to believe that our government would spend tens of millions of dollars on these kinds of silly pseudoscientific exercises, but this is the way it's done.

Then there's the question of determining how much damage is done to an average person who is exposed. What kind of a person? An old person? A baby? Someone who already has cancer or asthma? No, the assumption is that it's a white male between the ages of nineteen and thirty-eight who is employed and therefore eating well, and doesn't have any existing health problems. Based on that set of assumptions, we draw a numerical analysis that says okay, 0.6 is safe, 0.7 is dangerous. We're going to manage this thing so that you only get 0.6.

This is a numerical system. It excludes participation by the public. It's based on all kinds of faulty philosophical assumptions that are never mentioned in the discussion of a risk assessment. A person, often wearing a white lab coat, will come out and say, "Okay, the answer is 0.6 is safe, and if you don't like that, just because you want clean breast milk for your babies, it's up to you to prove that this stuff in your breast milk will harm your baby before we'll take any action." That is risk assessment, that is the way the system works. And that is why we have a totally polluted planet.

Closing the Loophole
of Uncertainty

Nancy Myers

Nancy Myers exudes a quiet determination and attentive precision that belie the fact that she has been a critical player in educating millions of people about issues of health, the environment, and peace. As communications director of the Science and Environmental Health Network (SEHN), she participated in the seminal 1998 Wingspread conference, which introduced the precautionary principle to public discourse in the United States.

As a writer and editor, she has been instrumental in offering the principle as a useful tool for activists and policymakers. She has published pithy fact sheets, arguments, statements, and articles including "Debating the Precautionary Principle," "Questions for Precautionary Thinking," and "The Precautionary Principle Puts Values First" (available on the SEHN website, www.sehn.org). She was a principal drafter of the founding statement of ecological medicine (see "Ecological Medicine: A Call for Inquiry and Action" at the back of this book).

Previously she served as managing editor of the Bulletin of the Atomic Scientists, *the "Doomsday Clock" magazine. As the Cold War ended, she developed some of the first international security writing fellowships for journalists from the former Soviet Union. She was executive director of the Educational Foundation for Nuclear Science from 1993 to 1997 and coedited, with George Lopez,* Peace and Security: The Next Generation. *She has both witnessed and participated in the growth of international civil society in recent decades.*

＊   ＊   ＊

NOW CONTRAST THE RISK ASSESSMENT MODEL with the precautionary principle, which dictates that when an activity raises threats of harm to human health or the environment, precautionary measures should be taken, even if some cause and effect relationships are not fully established scientifically.

What does that mean? It's science linked with values. The precautionary principle embodies a set of values. It requires certain values and ethics in the process of environmental decision making. What values does the precautionary principle embody? Protection of human health and environmental health. The public values of protecting the commons—that which we share with other species and other human beings—are elevated over private gain.

Protecting human health and protecting ecosystems are the same thing. They are interdependent, and the acknowledgment of that interdependence is a value that is embodied in the precautionary principle. Qualities such as respect, cooperation, and empathy are proper responses to this kind of interdependence.

Another value the precautionary principle embodies is attention to consequences and repercussions, which is at the heart of a precautionary approach. Precaution, in fact, is a translation of a German term that literally means "forecaring"—not just being cautious, but exercising foresight and care. It implies taking a longer view. These values don't stand alone in the precautionary principle. They underlie other concepts such as restoration, prevention, and sustainability.

The precautionary principle also exposes the values that prevail in current decision making, what we might call economics *über alles*. This mind-set has slipped into environmental decision making through a big loophole—the scientific uncertainty loophole—which holds that as long as there is some scientific uncertainty about the potential harm caused by something, there is no justification for preventing it. The precautionary principle closes this loophole.

A thorough alternatives assessment prevents us from arbitrarily narrowing the questions and the possibilities. It challenges the rigidity of rules that have limited the protection of health. It is another term for wisdom, a process that helps us ask bigger questions, take the longer view, and use our best judgment. These are the values embraced by people working on toxics issues, conservation, and ecosystem protection, and they're at the heart of the intent of many environmental laws. But even more than that, they represent the way that most people think human beings should behave. They're what we should have learned in kindergarten: to be kind and respectful and careful, to look before leaping, to be fair and to cooperate, and to be responsible. The precautionary principle extends these values to the natural world, not just to other human beings. It gives backbone to what we sense is right.

The precautionary principle keeps us on track, supplying a norm for making decisions that support and protect health. It applies this norm at the very spot where the decision-making process most often gets sidetracked: the misuse of science. Working to establish different norms for decision making than those that now prevail is hard, but we must learn to reflexively put health and the commons first, to look for repercussions, to shift burdens appropriately, to be inclusive and transparent in decision making, and to be open to better ways of doing things. The precautionary principle is an ideal tool to help us do that.

Putting Precaution on the Street

Martha Arguello

Dr. Martha Dina Arguello, raised in the rough streets of East Los Angeles, is an activist with twenty-five years' experience in social justice struggles in Southern California. In recent years she has become a dynamic force in the region's environmental justice movement, working as an environmental health coordinator with Physicians for Social Responsibility (PSR). She has expanded PSR's environmental health programs into the areas of pesticide reform, air quality, and environmental justice organizing, and has collaborated with the groundbreaking Health Care without Harm coalition.

There may be no one else whose work exemplifies more perfectly the fact that human rights and environmental health are mutually dependent. She has consistently shown that the struggles for social justice and environmental justice cannot be separated, and that by uniting them we can begin solving the problems of both. She serves on the boards or advisory groups of a number of organizations, including the Science and Environmental Health Network, the Steering Committee of Californians for Pesticide Reform, the Los Angeles Unified School District community pest-management team, and the Latino Issues Forum's water and energy advisory groups.

Most recently, she has joined forces with Carolyn Raffensperger and the Science and Environmental Health Network to bring the precautionary principle to Los Angeles, where she has achieved impressive results applying it to low-income communities and communities of color.

❀   ❀   ❀

I WAS BORN IN NICARAGUA and raised in Los Angeles, surrounded by gangs and violence. But I was able to emerge as an organizer. In fact, organizing saved my life. I came to doing environmental work after listening to a talk about breast milk contamination.

I had been a health advocate and worked with women with breast cancer, and I was having a growing sense of disquiet. In Spanish it's *inquietud*, a sort of anxious restlessness. I was trying to explain to younger and younger women why they were getting virulent breast cancers. In the midst of this disquiet, I heard Michael Lerner and Sandra Steingraber talk, and I had an epiphany, a moment that changed my life. All the strands of my life, the experiences of being in a gang, going to the University of California at Los Angeles, working in Nicaragua for the Sandinista government, all of it suddenly came together and I could feel a sense of purpose. I found a job very quickly with Physicians for Social Responsibility in Los Angeles.

One of the first things that was being talked about as I came on was the precautionary principle. There was a group of very forward-thinking community folks and a doctor from our organization who decided to put the precautionary principle in the preamble of this new integrated pest-management policy for the school district. It institutionalized several key aspects of the precautionary principle, including democratic participation, so that affected people got to sit at the table and make decisions along with the district staff. There were parents and community members, a physician, a nurse, and representatives from the environmental community.

When we first started talking about the principle, people said, "Well, that's a nice theory, but what is it really?" For a school district struggling with its pesticide use problem, it meant that we looked at the list of products they were using. Eighty-six percent of the school districts in California were using known reproductive toxins, known developmental toxins, and known carcinogens. Inordinate amounts of Roundup were being used in schools and are still being used in many school districts despite the Healthy Schools Act, which is supposed to offer less toxic integrated pest management options. If you have children in school districts in California, you have an absolute right to know what's being used and to be placed on a list so that the school will tell you.

We used the precautionary principle as a filter. We looked at the 135 products that the district had been using and asked, "Is it a known reproductive toxin? Is it a possible reproductive toxin? Is it a known carcinogen or possible carcinogen? Is it a developmental toxin, or a neurological toxin?" If it was known or probable or not known, it did not get on our approved list. We went from an approved list of 135 products, many containing highly toxic chemicals, to 32 products. That is how the precautionary principle works on the street.

Another key element is the promotion of alternatives. We had a group of ten people—parents, community members, environmentalists, former spray jockeys, and gardeners—sit down at a table and figure out how best to deal with our weed problem without using Roundup: everything from bringing goats to steam machines into the district. The coupling of innovation and having to use alternatives has made that policy work. It's not perfect. We have to be constantly on guard because institutions move slowly and they tend to revert to what they know, and what they know is to spray.

The story of how all this came to be in Los Angeles is interesting. A mother dropping off her children at school saw two men in hazmat (hazardous materials) suits spraying right near the school stairs. As her children walked through the mist of pesticide, one of them turned around and said, "Mommy, it really tastes awful." This mother, Rubina, a very unreasonable woman, called many people including Pesticide Watch and other organizations. That was the birth of the new policy. It took a year from the time Rubina's children were sprayed to the time that the policy passed. It has now been three years, and the district staff, including former spray jockeys, have been recognized across the country for the cutting-edge work that they've done. This is the power of implementing the precautionary principle, and the power of one concerned individual.

In January 2002, we organized one of the first precautionary principle workshops on the West Coast. It was one of the most ethnically diverse events any of us had ever been to in Los Angeles. Three months later, California passed a very strong law implementing environmental justice policies and requiring that all policies and programs be fair to all communities, regardless of income level and race. This initiated a process in which panels of experts and community members in broad representation, including industry, will be reviewing all the plans for each California EPA department, from the Air District to the Department of Pesticide Regulation to the Waste Management Board. We are seeing the power of theory and practice come together in the precautionary principle. Amazing things are happening in California. In the face of the many rollbacks at the national level, California remains forward-thinking and is figuring out ways to implement precaution, but it needs your support to persevere.

But What Is the Alternative?

Mary O'Brien

Mary O'Brien has that special kind of quirky brilliance that shifts our perception of the world a few degrees and gives us new eyes. She is a trained listener and meticulous observer of both the natural world and people. She never hesitates to press the thorny questions that challenge our most basic assumptions. Her heart has perfect pitch for the well-being of all life, especially that of nonhuman beings. By uniting these traits, she has become a formidable force in the field of ecological medicine.

Until recently, she served as the ecosystem projects director of the Science and Environmental Health Network, where she applied her keen powers of contemplation to the question of what the precautionary principle means for ecosystem health. She is one of the nation's leading specialists in ecosystem science, ecological restoration, alternatives to pushing humans and other species to the brink with flawed "risk assessment" strategies, and the ramifications and implications of the precautionary principle for living systems. From her base in her beloved southwestern Oregon, she has also served as a staff scientist for the Northwest Coalition for Alternatives to Pesticides, the Environmental Law Alliance Worldwide, the Environmental Research Foundation, and the Hells Canyon Preservation Council. She is the author of Making Better Environmental Decisions: An Alternative to Risk Assessment.

*   *   *

A PRECAUTIONARY APPROACH to ecosystems implies that when an activity or condition raises credible threats of harm to ecosystems, precautionary measures should be taken, even if cause and effect relationships are not fully established. But ecosystems today are faced not only with harm from proximate physical or chemical activities or conditions such as overharvesting, fire suppression, highways, global warming, and chemical and genetic pollution. They also face harm from certain human laws, rules, policies, and institutional conditions, such as the privatization of water supplies, World Trade Organization regulations, the legal protection of corporate profit at all costs, and the release of genetically engineered life forms.

Whether we're talking of precautionary measures in relation to harm from physical activity or from social organizations, public consideration of alternatives to the potentially harmful activities or arrangements is essential. Because of the complexity of ecosystems and the multiplicity of sources of harm to them, precautionary measures often require large social changes that can feel threatening, not only to corporations that profit by causing ecosystem harm, or to agencies that have become habituated to permitting harm, but also to individuals who have become financially or psychologically tied to work, leisure, or consumptive practices that degrade the ecosystem.

I want to tell a story that illustrates the importance of defending our ability to even consider alternatives. Where I live in Eugene, the Oregon Department of Transportation is proposing that a four-lane bypass highway called West Eugene Parkway be built through the last 0.1 percent of wetland prairie and upland prairie remaining in the 100-mile-long Willamette Valley, which extends from Eugene to Portland. When white settlers came to Oregon, one-third of the valley was covered with wetland upland prairie. In the last hundred years, 99.9 percent of this wetland upland prairie has been drained, farmed, developed, or paved over. Moreover, the remaining tiny wetland upland prairie in West Eugene through which the highway would be constructed is Bureau of Land Management park land, bought with national taxpayers' money for conservation through our nation's Land and Water Conservation Fund. On top of that, a butterfly, federally listed as endangered, and the plant its larvae must eat, also federally listed as threatened, and a daisy, federally listed as endangered, all grow in and/or next to the route of the proposed highway. The highway would be 92 meters wide, as wide as a football field is long.

I attended a University of Oregon teach-in during which approximately 1,000 University of Oregon students and Eugene residents listened to five university professors talk about various problems associated with a U.S. invasion of Iraq. One of these, a physics professor, showed how our current 60 percent dependence on imported oil is accounted for almost entirely by transportation habits, such as the fact that the average American drives 15,000 miles a year in a vehicle that averages only 30 miles per gallon of gas on highways such as the proposed West Eugene Parkway.

Clearly the West Eugene Parkway is a classic case in which alternatives are available and essential in order to avert global oil wars, avoid extinction of wetlands species, prevent the fragmentation of a wondrous and rare ecosystem, and substitute walkable, livable neighborhoods for highway-dependent sprawl.

In 1988, the Oregon Department of Transportation had proposed a similar western bypass highway in Portland. In response, a citizen organization called 1,000 Friends of Oregon initiated an alternative that featured some roadway construction, neighborhood and urban transit-oriented developments, light rail, express buses, local feeder buses, and bicycle and pedestrian improvements. Compared to the bypass, this alternative reduced vehicle trips, cost less to construct, reduced energy consumption and emissions of air pollutants and greenhouse gases, and reduced highway congestion by 18 percent. Eventually the Oregon Department of Transportation agreed that this was the better alternative, and it was adopted and implemented.

Similarly, coalitions of individuals and organizations in Eugene are currently working on developing alternatives to the West Eugene Parkway. The parkway would be a federally funded highway, and all federally funded projects—whether forest logging, pesticide spraying, or the building of a military facility—must be analyzed in an environmental impact statement that is written according to the regulations of the National Environmental Policy Act (NEPA). The most important single legal requirement within these NEPA regulations is that when a project that may have a significant environmental impact is proposed, "All reasonable alternatives must be considered and fully analyzed for their potential impacts." There is no clearer and more wonderful U.S. law requiring the consideration of alternatives to health or ecosystem-threatening activities than NEPA. As the NEPA regulation itself states, "This section, i.e. requiring consideration of alternatives, is the heart of the Environmental Impact Statement, sharply defining the issues, and providing a clear basis for choice among options by the decision maker and the public."

Of course, this issue extends beyond NEPA. Consideration of reasonable alternatives is always at the heart of taking precautionary measures within ecosystems and public health situations. In other words, when an activity or condition raises credible threats of harm to public health or ecosystems, we cannot take precautionary measures if we don't consider alternatives.

On October 2, 2002, however, a bipartisan group of senators introduced into Congress a highway and transit bill called the MEGA Stream Act (House bill F.3031). MEGA Stream stands for "maximum economic growth for America through environmental streamlining." It gives the secretary of transportation the final authority to decide whether any alternatives to a proposed federally funded highway or transit project will be considered. The secretary could now say, "My highway project will be the only considered, and no one can suggest an alternative. Analysis of my project will not consider the following possible environmental impacts," and then could list them.

In other words, our nation's citizens would be prevented from proposing precautionary measures on highway and transit decisions. This follows by weeks the introduction of a similar bill that would eliminate consideration of any alternatives in proposals for logging of the nation's public forests to supposedly prevent forest fires. It is a fundamental corporate attack on NEPA. It is not unlike the General Agreement on Tariffs and Trade (GATT) and other free-trade agreements, including those of the World Trade Organization, that eliminate the ability of a sovereign nation to refuse genetically engineered food or products made by slave labor, or to favor products that have been produced in an economically or socially respectful manner.

This is a concerted effort to limit citizens' and even nations' ability to be precautionary and suggest alternatives. The MEGA Stream Act is based on the idea that both the consideration of alternatives and environmental impact analysis get in the way of maximum economic growth. The powerful bipartisan senate sponsors of the bill are right. Wetlands sometimes get in the way of developers. Spotted owls sometimes get in the way of logging companies. Democracy, when it's alive, often gets in the way of corporations and individuals who would buy and sell the earth, drain it, log it, desertify it, homogenize it, tear it up, erode it, poison it, genetically engineer it, or cook it. In the end, it may be that the most efficient, tyrannical, and effective method of preventing implementation of the precautionary principle by our communities or any nation is to simply legally prohibit us from considering alternatives to destructive practices.

The consideration of alternatives is the heart of an environmental impact statement and of precautionary principle implementation. Prevent consideration of alternatives and you have taken away the precautionary principle. This means we must create and defend social and legal frameworks that allow and even require those who would rather keep their heads firmly in the sand to look around and to look decent alternatives in the eye.

Part III

Public Health, Cancer, and Prevention

Reconciling Human Rights, Public Health, and the Web of Life

Ted Schettler

ADVANCES IN SCIENTIFIC UNDERSTANDING, new and improved treatments for disease based on new technologies, and public health successes during the twentieth century have certainly lengthened life and reduced morbidity and mortality from specific diseases. However, a new pattern of human disease has emerged that is not being adequately addressed by our medical system. In fact, we have in many ways seen a deterioration of our public health infrastructure. If we extend our lens further, we find that there's been a real deterioration in the ecosystems around us. Ecological medicine is an attempt to address these realities.

What is ecological medicine? As we move from a consideration of only the individual in contemporary medical practice to the public health perspective and then to the ecological perspective, we actually move through an expansion of constituencies, and expansion of ethical considerations, and a growth of ethical complexity. Medical practitioners advocate for individual people. Public health institutions advocate for the public, for communities and populations of people, and look at social, environmental, and economic factors as they have a direct impact on the health of people. Ecological medicine goes further in that it does not focus only on the health of humans to the exclusion of other species and ecosystems.

In conventional medical practice, ethical concerns are largely centered on the rights of individual people and the obligation of practitioners to provide competent care with compassion. I took a little journey through the statements of ethics of the American Medical Association, of some state medical associations, and of the Public Health Association. What you find in the American

Medical Association's statement is the right to competent care and respect, the right to know and the right to choice. The physician is charged to be competent, to obey the law, and to seek changes in legal requirements that are contrary to the best interest of the patient. The physician is also to contribute to the improvement of the community and the betterment of public health. There's a little bit of movement away from a total focus on the individual, but the principles explicitly state that while caring for a patient, the individual patient is of paramount concern.

Public health ethics more directly encounter the tension between what is best for individuals and what is best for communities and populations of people. A number of ethical traditions and concepts are relevant to public health ethics—communitarianism, civil liberties, human rights, and social justice, for example. From the communitarian perspective, public health ethics are based on the recognition that individual liberty and indeed human existence rely heavily on the interdependent and overlapping communities to which all of us belong—families, neighborhoods, and religious and other social groups.

The exclusive pursuit of private interest erodes the network of social environments on which we all depend. The ability of an individual to practice autonomy depends on the active maintenance of the institutions of civil society, where citizens learn respect for others as well as self-respect, and where a community is dependent on the contribution of its members to shared projects. The relationship of private and public interest involves a mesh of complementary and reciprocal rights and responsibilities. A spirit of solidarity provides voice and support for those who are less fortunate. Here we see tensions begin to arise between individual and public interest. Social justice concerns might require a maximization of return from limited social resources. There may be conflicting views about what is in a child's best interest, or the interests of future generations.

The American Public Health Association Code of Ethics starts out by saying that public health should principally address the fundamental causes of disease and the requirements to prevent adverse health outcomes. Public health should achieve community health in a way that respects the rights of individuals. Public health policies, programs, and priorities should be developed and evaluated through processes that ensure an opportunity for input from all community members. The code then goes on to address the empowerment of disenfranchised people; respect for diverse values, beliefs, and cultures; confidentiality; and professional competence.

One principle begins hesitantly to step outside that framework. It says that public health programs and policies should be implemented in a manner that most enhances the physical and social environment. It seems obvious that people and their physical environment are interdependent. People depend upon the resources of their natural and constructed environments for life. A damaged or unbalanced natural environment and a constructed environment of poor design or in poor condition will have an adverse effect on the health of people. Conversely, people can have a profound effect on their natural environment through consumption of resources and generation of waste. So the official documents of public health point to a bigger picture.

That's where we get into ecological medicine, which extends its concerns beyond humans to include other species and the physical and spiritual world more generally. Ecological medicine focuses even more on relationships, and it encounters even more fundamental ethical tensions. Here, we are concerned about our relationships not only with each other, but with other species, landscapes, and ecosystems. A human rights perspective suddenly seems narrow. Some people make efforts to extend the reach of a rights-based approach to other species and ecosystems, but a rights-based approach is one of contracts and negotiations. Historically it is based on language and reason, and organisms that can't speak the language of rights don't get to sit at this negotiating table.

The talk of a need for an environmental or ecological ethic is not new. In 1949, Aldo Leopold wrote, "An ethic, ecologically, is a limitation on freedom of action." He then immediately introduced the notion of restraint: "In the struggle for existence, ethics dealt first with the relation between individuals, later with the relation between individual and society. The extension of ethics to land is an evolutionary possibility and an ecological necessity. All ethics so far evolved rest upon a single premise that the individual is a member of a community of interdependent parts. A person's instincts prompt him to compete for a place in the community, but his ethics prompt him to cooperate. The land ethic simply enlarges the boundaries of the community to include soils, waters, plants and animals, or collectively, the land." But this makes ethical tensions become more pronounced. This is not just about the competing interests of individual people and human communities. Now the framework has expanded to include all communities. It takes the human out of the center of the universe.

One understanding of a genuinely ecological medicine is that individual components of an ecological system and the system as a whole exist in a dialectic relationship. The whole is contingent upon and reciprocates with its components, and with the greater whole of which it is a part. Whole and parts coevolve. Cause becomes effect; effect become cause. Even human rights, based on the inherent worth and dignity of individuals, exist within a complex set of relationships. In fact, it is precisely this set of relationships that defines the individual. Without relationships, individuals do not exist. But a fundamental dilemma that then arises out of this dialectic relationship between individuals and the larger system is how to identify where the individual begins and ends. The physical, biological, and social sciences show how blurred the boundaries really are. Individual people exist only in relationship with larger communities that include people, fungi, bacteria, plants, animals, forests, farms, and cities.

Ecological medicine must rest on an ethical framework that bears witness to and acknowledges the tensions inherent in this expanded perspective. Reconciliation of these tensions may not be desirable or plausible. Tensions are inherent in any ecological system; they give the system shape and help create the conditions for systemwide health. Too much force on one side breaks the tension. Resilience is lost. Resilience is essential to a healthy system.

An ethic of ecological medicine will recognize the voice of the individual person, the voice of human communities, and the voice of other-than-human communities. Ecological medicine recognizes interdependence and the dialectic relationships inherent in ecosystems. But it does not depend solely on human health concerns as the basis for forming relationships within a larger ecological perspective. Ecological medicine seeks to put human rights in a broader perspective. Ecological medicine is based on respectful relationships with humans, other species, and the natural world more generally. But beyond respect, it is based on an ethic of care and reciprocity.

What might this mean in practice? We are only at the earliest stages of this movement, but we can see the direction in which we need to go. For health care providers, there needs to be a real modification of the professional ethic to include a larger awareness of public health and the environmental impacts of medical practices. Life cycle analyses of the materials used in health care are required. Purchasing, use, and disposal choices should be based on a deeper understanding of the long-term impacts on the larger ecosystem.

Health care providers and public health professionals need to learn to run decisions through an ethical screen—a screen not only of rights, but also of respect, caring, and reciprocity. Is a practice respectful of life and relationships? Whose life, what life, what relationships? Even more fundamental and more challenging, we need to individually and collectively examine our attitudes toward death and dying—the measures we take to prolong human life and the impacts of life-extending technologies as they reverberate broadly through ecosystems.

Perhaps most important, all of us—parents, children, students, and medical professionals—need to learn how to feel compassionate and caring toward the earth and all its inhabitants, so that we respond to the sight of a dead or dying river as we would at the bedside of a dead or dying sister.

Florence Nightingale:
Mystic, Visionary, Healer

Barbara Dossey

Barbara Dossey, Ph.D., R.N., H.N.C., F.A.A.N., is a legend in the field of holistic nursing, a discipline she helped invent. She has been internationally recognized and widely honored for her countless contributions toward elevating the nursing profession to its rightful stature as a keystone of health care. She has authored or coauthored an astounding nineteen books, including, most recently, her definitive Florence Nightingale: Mystic, Visionary, and Healer.

Nightingale is Barbie's personal "shero," and almost any conversation with Barbie inevitably turns to Nightingale. She has good reason to feel this way, because the nineteenth-century nurse was arguably medicine's greatest visionary as far as public health and the role of nursing are concerned.

Barbie assembled many of the basic textbooks used by nurses around the world, including the American Holistic Nurses' Association's Holistic Nursing: A Handbook for Practice *and the American Association of Clinical Nursing's* Handbook of Critical Care Nursing, *as well as* Rituals of Healing. *She is a fellow of the American Academy of Nursing, its most prestigious honor, and has received countless other honors and awards, including the venerated American Journal of Nursing Book of the Year Award (seven times!), the Holistic Nurse of the Year Award from the American Holistic Nurses' Association, and the designation Healer of the Year from the Nurse Healers' Professional Associates International. She is currently director of Holistic Nursing Consultants in Santa Fe, New Mexico.*

In the long struggle to humanize health care beyond the narrow boundaries mainstream medicine has imposed, Barbie has tirelessly sought to resacralize the healing profession. In this process, it is nurses who have often led the way. It comes as no surprise that Nightingale's legacy would resonate with her, because no one else comes as close to carrying Nightingale's socially and spiritually engaged healing tradition into the twenty-first century.

❦ ❦ ❦

IF WE ARE GOING TO HEAL our failing health care system, it behooves us to reflect on our medical history. One of the figures in that history we can learn a great deal from and be inspired by is Florence Nightingale, whose name nearly everyone has heard, but whose contributions have been largely forgotten or misunderstood.

Nightingale was born in 1820 and died in 1910. She is given credit for starting secular nursing. She insisted that everyone, including the poor, should have access to health care. Anyone who came into St. Thomas Hospital, where she started the first school of nursing in 1860, could be treated regardless of religious persuasion or social status.

Florence Nightingale's mother, Fanny Smith, was said to be one of the most beautiful women in all of England. Her father, William Edward Nightingale, was an honest politician who refused to bribe the electorate and who decided, after he lost an election, to home-school his two daughters. Her parents were wealthy, refined, and highly educated people with large estates, so Nightingale received a classical Cambridge home education. She literally got what we today would consider a postdoctoral education. She was fluent in five foreign languages: Greek, Latin, French, German, and Italian. She studied advanced mathematics in her twenties. One of her aunts, realizing how bright she was, had insisted that Florence's father allow her to have advanced mathematics lessons, something highly unusual for a young woman at the time, and she was tutored by one of the leading mathematicians in England.

From a young age, Florence was interested in why people were ill. When the family would travel, she would keep diaries, observing and reflecting upon who was sick in different towns and cities and why. She was a prolific writer. She left 14,000 letters in her archives, the largest such private collection in a British library. She left over 100 huge documents, some 2,000 — 3,000 pages long, and over 20 books. Her most famous book, *Notes on Nursing*, has been in publication ever since it was written in 1860, and has been translated into many languages. Most everything that we would like to see in modern health care, Nightingale wrote about in *Notes on Nursing*, including partnerships and complementary and alternative therapies. Her work is as profoundly relevant as ever. She was a century ahead of her time. By the time of her death there were 1,000 Nightingale training programs in the United States alone, and her direct influence via her nursing program and training extended to 20 countries.

Nightingale's observations of public health led her to emphasize the six Ds—dirt, drink, diet, damp, drafts, and drains—as the main factors in illness in her time. Drink, of course, related to excessive alcohol consumption, but also referred to polluted water. Nightingale had literally revolutionized the world's health care system by the end of her lifetime.

What is less known about Florence Nightingale today is that she was an inspired mystic. She was also highly rational and devoted to rigorous scientific research. As a multilingual scholar, she read spiritual texts critically. She really didn't like the fact that the feminine metaphor had been left out of the Bible, for example. This woman was way ahead of her time. She would look at the miracles and scribble in her Bible, "A very important story, no scientific fact." She was a very complex, multidimensional genius who would get flashes of intuition. She decided suddenly, for example, that the whole British Army needed to be reorganized, and that there needed to be a discipline called professional nursing to parallel the advances in the medical profession. Then she just went ahead and got it done. She had an extraordinary ability to accomplish enormous tasks, but in her letters, she often reprimands herself for not accomplishing as much as she should. This is a mystic's interpretation of how she is leading her life. The closer Nightingale gets to the Divine, the more she sees her own imperfections.

By age thirty, Nightingale was fully equipped to go out in the world. She told her father, "You have no son. I choose not to marry. I need an allowance," and he acquiesced. She took her cook, her maid, her messenger, and her footman to London with her and became the superintendent of a small twenty-seven-bed hospital for distressed governesses, which she completely reorganized. Within one year, she was called out to be the superintendent of nurses at a giant British military hospital in Turkey. She was thrust in to the very bloody Crimean War of 1854—1856.

She experienced a clear calling to help humanity discover forms of organization that would permit people to live in harmony with God's purposes. During the war she often had to deal with literally four and five and six thousand wounded soldiers, many of whom were lying in the hallways of enormous barracks, and figure out how to take care of them. When she returned to England she outlined clearly for Queen Victoria what was wrong not only with the army in Turkey, but the army throughout the whole British Empire. She told Victoria that if she did not get rid of the six Ds—the dirt, drink, draft, drains, damp, and atrocious diet—and improve health conditions, including the health of those in the surrounding villages, and, especially, educate women, she would have a sick army. She understood the importance of what we now call the environment, both physical and socioeconomic. She was a pioneer of holistic medical thinking.

Nightingale made only two public appearances from the age of thirty-seven to the age of ninety, but she became world famous. She knew how to make the most of her time and how to focus her energy. She worked with Sidney Herbert, the secretary at war, for five years to reorganize the British Army's medical department, explaining how to build drains, latrines, and healthier buildings. She worked with the leading medical statistician of the day, Dr. William Farr. She was one of the first people to explode the pie chart and to add color to highlight a diagram in reports to the queen and the parliament. She was a passionate statistician—all of her work in applied statistics is profound. She proved that most British deaths in the Crimean War were caused by poor sanitation. Nightingale never went to India, but she was the person most knowledgeable about the health of the British Army in India. No routine medical records were kept at the time, so she created a medical records form and sent it directly to all the army encampments in India. Because Nightingale was famous, the forms would be sent directly back with all the requested data. Henry Dunant, the Swiss man who started the International Red Cross, gave Nightingale all the credit for having inspired its creation through her work in Turkey and in the Crimea. She never wavered in pursuing her goals and in her singleminded devotion to spreading health awareness to the four corners of the earth.

Nightingale was an extraordinarily effective, prophetic health visionary and force of nature. In a 1893 essay, she summed up her hopes for the future with words that are as relevant and resonant now as they were then:

> In the future, which I shall not see, for I am old, may a better way be opened. May the methods by which every infant, every human being will have the best chance at health, the methods by which every sick person will have the best chance of discovery, be learned and practiced. Hospitals are only an intermediate stage of civilization, never intended at all events to take in the whole sick population. Hospitals should do people no harm. May we hope that every nurse will be an atom in the hierarchy of the ministries of the highest . . . not alone . . . but being part of the whole. High hopes shall not be deceived.

Reversing the Cancer Epidemic

Samuel Epstein

Dr. Samuel Epstein has bravely exposed one of the greatest scandals of the twentieth century: the tragic failure of the war on cancer and the concerted effort by the cancer establishment to prevent prevention. He was among the first to break this news, which he did in 1978 with his landmark book The Politics of Cancer.

After beginning his career as a laboratory chief documenting the metabolic origins of cancer, he impeccably documented the direct effects of industrial chemicals as causes of cancer. He wrote the original proposal for what became the Toxic Substances Control Act of 1976. He charged that industrial interests had conspired to deflect, distort, or even destroy evidence of the carcinogenicity of specific compounds, especially when profitable products were at stake. His straightforward conclusion: "While much is known about the science of cancer, its prevention depends largely, if not exclusively, on political action."

Today a professor of occupational and environmental medicine at the University of Illinois at Chicago, Sam Epstein is a direct heir to Rachel Carson, whose chilling exposé The Silent Spring *first alerted the nation and the world to the health horrors of DDT and industrial pollution. As with Rachel Carson, his courageous public warning has drawn fierce fire. It landed him on a White House hit list during the Reagan era, and efforts were made to keep him off any government committees studying cancer prevention. An actual smoking-gun memo read, "Get him out. Horrible."*

Conversely, in 1998 he was honored with the Right Livelihood Award, known as the "alternative Nobel Prize." He has written innumerable scientific articles and several compelling books, including The Safe Shopper's Bible, *which details avoidable carcinogens in consumer products. He is the chairman of the Cancer Prevention Coalition, a global network of scientists, public servants, and activists.*

✿   ✿   ✿

THERE ARE TWO VERY IMPORTANT REASONS why you should take an interest in cancer prevention and the present cancer epidemic: One in every two men and one in every three women will get cancer in your lifetime, and most of these cancers are avoidable. We are failing to avoid them because of a complex of scientific, political, financial, and public policy considerations.

But there is an even more important reason to pay attention to this crisis. Many people share passionate concerns about issues such as human rights, social justice, and corporate globalization. However, these are not issues around which you can readily organize grassroots national campaigns. You're simply not going to fire up 250 million Americans or every single family in this country about such issues, however important they are. The only way to succeed is on the basis of an appeal to self-interest. You can go out into the community and the whole nation and say to all citizens, "You or some of your family members are going to get cancer, and a substantial number will die from cancers, most of which could be avoided." You then stand a realistic chance of creating a powerful grassroots national campaign.

In the latter part of the twentieth century, we've seen the emergence of three runaway industrial technologies that have threatened not only our country but the totality of the environment. The first are the petrochemical and agrichemical industries. These started in the 1940s, when industry first learned how to synthesize new chemicals, which had never existed before, by fractional distillation of petroleum and by molecular splicing. The second is nuclear technology, and the third and most recent is genetic engineering. In this connection, I should mention that most of the public, and many scientists, are under the impression that genetic engineering products are just appearing on the market. In fact, we've been exposed to genetically engineered milk since 1985, when milk from unpublicized large-scale national production trials conducted by Monsanto, working with captive land grant universities, was sold to an unsuspecting and uninformed public. Since then, the sale of rBGH milk has become widespread in this country. About 10 percent of cows are injected with genetically modified bovine growth hormone, and this milk is bulked with nonhormonal milk, thus contaminating all the nation's milk, with the exception of that of a few socially responsible dairy companies.

Cancer is the only disease for which we have absolute trend data on incidence and mortality for the last few decades. Certainly we are concerned about a wide range of other problems—reproductive, immunological, neurological, and respiratory—but we don't have as solid incidence and mortality data for them as we do for cancer. Most carcinogens—chemicals and agents that produce cancer—also produce a very wide range of these other effects. In that sense, cancer is a paradigm or broad indicator of the adverse impacts of toxic chemicals in our environment. Moreover, cancer is the only major adverse impact for which we can clearly relate a direct causal relationship between avoidable carcinogenic exposures and escalating trends. Cancer is thus a quantifiable manifestation of runaway industrial technologies that affect all of us.

Cancer is also an expression of corporate crime and regulatory complicity, social injustice, the denial of the right to know, and a massive failure of the democratic decision-making process.

What are the facts of the cancer epidemic? The incidence and mortality rates have escalated dramatically since the 1940s. Since 1950, there's been about a 55 percent overall increase in all cancer rates. When broken down to particular cancers, excluding lung cancer (which is largely related to smoking), the majority of the increases since 1950 have been nonsmoking cancers. This doesn't mean that smoking isn't the single most important cause of all cancers, which it certainly is. But the non—smoking related cancers are largely an expression of involuntary and avoidable exposures to carcinogens in our air, water, food and other consumer products, soil, and the workplace.

For example, testicular cancer is up 100 percent; for men between 28 and 35, the incidence has gone up by 300 percent. Adult brain cancer: 80 percent. Breast cancer and male colon cancer: 60 percent. Childhood cancers: 20 percent. Brain and nervous system cancers in children: 40 percent.

What are the causes of the epidemic? Contrary to what industry and the cancer establishment—the National Cancer Institute (NCI) and American Cancer Society (ACS)—tell us, it's not the fact that people are living longer. The incidence figures are age standardized, or adjusted to reflect the increasing longevity of the population. What we've seen in children is a perfect example. The very high increase in childhood cancer makes it clear we're not dealing with problems of longevity.

Smoking is responsible for about a quarter of the increase in all cancer rates, but we also have clear evidence there are other important causes of lung cancer, particularly air pollution, radon, and a wide range of occupational exposures. In addition, while vast amounts of money are being spent on genetic research, genetics has virtually nothing at all to do with the escalating cancer incidence. Genetics is responsible for perhaps 5 to 6 percent of breast cancers, and about 1 percent of all colon cancers. In no way could the genetics of the human population have changed in the last few decades; that takes millennia.

Dietary fat, often named as a key factor in cancer, is not in itself necessarily a cause, though high-fat diets are clearly bad from the point of view of heart disease. It's what's *in the fat* that matters, the contamination by pesticides and industrial chemicals that concentrate in fatty tissues in animals fed in feedlots in the highly industrialized countries and that rise up the food chain. In southern Mediterranean countries, where olive oil is in constant use and the diet consists of as much as 40 to 45 percent fat, there are very low cancer rates.

There's overwhelming evidence that the increase in cancer rates results from avoidable exposures to carcinogens in the workplace, in consumer products, and in air, water, and soil. First, there's a vast body of analytical or body burden chemical data. If you examine the fat in your own body or in fish and wildlife, you'll find some two or three hundred industrial chemicals and carcinogens. Even in the Arctic, where there is no industry to speak of, we find PCBs and other carcinogenic and toxic chemicals.

Animal studies are most important. There's substantial evidence from tests in mice and rats that clearly shows that many of these chemicals induce cancers, in many cases in the same sites as in humans. One example is DES, diethylstilbestrol. From 1938 to 1950, there were about twenty different animal studies that clearly demonstrated that this synthetic estrogenic chemical was a major cause of reproductive cancers, even at the lowest levels tested. Yet in the mid-1950s, obstetricians and gynecologists were giving it to women in unsubstantiated attempts to reduce complications of pregnancy and telling them it was perfectly safe. The animal evidence didn't faze them. "We don't have any human data," they protested. You know the rest of the story: DES caused cancers and birth deformities.

However, I must caution those who share my concerns about animal rights. Animal testing of chemicals, in the view of the independent scientific community, is the most reliable and only way of creating the strongest index of suspicion that the same chemicals will induce cancer in humans. We have a very strong body of human epidemiological data that has confirmed the significance of the animal data. However, I recognize that this is an unpopular and painful dilemma.

We also have epidemiological studies in fish and wildlife, called epizootics. We find fish in certain parts of the world with a very high incidence of tumors that we can relate to contaminated waters. Then there are the human studies: the occupational studies, the cancer clusters in certain communities, and the overall trends in industrialized nations versus nonindustrialized nations.

What has been happening to our ability to treat and cure cancers over all this time? In the 1960s, there was about a 49 percent five-year survival rate. Forty-nine percent of people survived five years after diagnosis in the 1960s, when virtually no money was being spent in these areas. Now, after billions of dollars have been poured into cancer treatment, the length of survival is about six years. It has barely increased over the last forty years for the great majority of common cancers in the overall population.

When it comes to the nonwhite population, the survival rate was 38 percent four decades ago and remains 38 percent today. So, although you read about alleged miracle cures, the great advances we're supposed to be making in treatment, if you look at the actual figures, the improvement over decades has been minimal, if any.

How does all this square up with what we are constantly hearing about these miracle cancer drugs? The answer lies in a deceptive statistical ploy. The efficacy of cancer drugs is determined on the basis of what we call tumor response. If a patient with cancer takes a drug and at the end of six months the tumor has shrunk in size, that's a tumor response. That's supposedly fine. We're doing very well indeed. Let's go out and market this miracle drug. Let's go out and make millions and billions out of it. However, if you follow up with these patients who have had a tumor response at six months after diagnosis and treatment, in twelve to eighteen months you generally find that the original tumor has recurred and often grown larger. Sometimes, the *treated* patient will die sooner than the *untreated* patient—and this is quite apart from the fact that the treated patient's quality of life is often devastated by highly toxic chemotherapy and radiation.

For the majority of cancer chemotherapeutic agents, there is questionable evidence of efficacy. There are some relatively rare cancers for which there is strong evidence of efficacy; for childhood cancer, where treatment is successful, the incidence of long-term recurrences are very high. Delayed toxic complications such as neurological, behavioral, and reproductive problems are also common, and the incidence of secondary cancers caused by the treatment itself is very high.

So much for the claimed advances in our ability to treat and cure cancer. Who is responsible for this public policy travesty? In 1971, President Nixon declared the war on cancer. He was persuaded by the leaders of the cancer establishment that if we could put a man on the moon, we could cure cancer in our lifetime. The budget of the National Cancer Institute in 1971 was about $200 million. It's now about $2 billion. The ACS, the largest private charity in the world, has an annual budget of well over $500 million. These budgets have escalated from relatively small amounts twenty or thirty years ago as the public has been assured that we will have the ability to treat and cure cancer if given more funding, when in fact the statistics say otherwise.

The cancer establishment consists of the NCI, ACS, and a national network of comprehensive cancer centers in major universities and hospitals all over the country. Their assets and resources are overwhelming. Apart from massive financial resources, they have major influence on the media through well-financed public relations campaigns that blanket the country.

The cancer establishment is fixated overwhelmingly on damage control:

screening, diagnosis, and treatment, and also genetic research. It displays virtual indifference, if not hostility, to cancer prevention. At the National Cancer Institute, for instance, occupational cancer, the single most important avoidable cancer, which we estimate is responsible for nearly 20 percent of all cancer
deaths in this country, receives about 1 percent of the budget. Cancer among
people of color, for which the rates are high, receives 1 percent of the budget.

The ACS has a long track record of actual hostility to cancer prevention.
It fought against the Delaney Amendment, which says, "Thou shalt not add
any level of carcinogens to food." It issued joint statements of support with
the Chlorine Institute saying there's no evidence that organochlorine pesticides represent any hazard whatsoever. A few years ago, just before PBS was
getting ready to air a program called *Pesticides in Our Children's Food,* a script
was somehow leaked. Actually, it was stolen from the desk of Marty Coughan,
the program director, and found its way to a PR operation with close ties to
the ACS. Immediately, memoranda were sent out to all regional ACS divi-
sions calling on them to contact the media and trivialize concerns about the
risks of infant and childhood foods being laced with carcinogenic pesticides.

The cancer establishment has further failed to inform Congress, regulatory agencies, and the public about the wide range of avoidable cancer risks.
Most cancers are largely avoidable, and we have very specific information on
the causes of a wide range of these cancers, such as breast, ovarian, and childhood cancers, as well as non-Hodgkins lymphoma.

What are the reasons for these distorted policies of the cancer establishment? They're twofold. They're an expression of a professional mind-set that
is fixated on damage control: diagnosis, treatment, and genetic research. This
arena is where the leaders come from and what they are interested in. But there
are also deep, interlocking conflicts of interest between the cancer establishment and the cancer drug, mammography, and other industries. This is most
obvious in relation to the ACS, but even a previous director of the National
Cancer Institute admitted in an unusually candid moment that the NCI has
become a "governmental pharmaceutical company."

One example is Taxol, a drug used in the treatment of ovarian and certain
other cancers. The basic research on it was done at the NCI with taxpayers'

money, your money. The moment it looked profitable, the NCI turned it over to Bristol-Myers Squibb, which manufactures the drug for about twenty cents for each five-milligram capsule, which it then sells for $5. So, the public has to pay twice? First, we pay for the research by funding the NCI to the tune of $4.6 billion annually. Then, we pay exorbitantly again for the same drug once it becomes marketable.

There used to be a fair pricing clause, a law that said that when drugs and useful products are developed by government, if they are turned over to industry, there have to be restrictions on industry's profits. However, the previous director of the National Institutes of Health, Harold Varmus, who has been the recipient of millions of dollars of funds from industry and the cancer establishment, said the fair pricing clause was a blow against industrial innovation, and he struck it down. So now industry can charge whatever it likes for drugs that you and I as taxpayers have funded.

The ties between the NCI and the mammography industry are even closer. Apart from these sorts of highly questionable arrangements, the ACS is the only charity in this country that funds political parties, which is supposedly illegal. According to the *Chronicle of Philanthropy*, the leading national watchdog of charities, "The American Cancer Society is more interested in accumulating wealth than saving lives."

In addition, both the ACS and NCI have maintained a policy over the last few decades of harassing practitioners of alternative and complementary medicine on the grounds that there's no evidence of efficacy or effectiveness. The overriding irony is that for the majority of the uses of toxic chemotherapy, there isn't significant evidence of increased survival rates. However, different standards are used for conventional versus alternative or complementary therapies. At the same time, the cancer establishment has, until very recently, denied public funds for development of trials for alternative or complementary therapy.

Running deep through all of this chicanery is a pattern of corporate and white-collar crime that is well documented. It is inextricably linked with decision making at the regulatory agency level, and it is linked with the policies and priorities of the ACS and NCI. In 1978, I had the privilege of drafting legislation for Congress on white-collar crime in the area of public health, which I defined as "crimes of economic motivation with public health consequences." Congressman John Conyers, Jr., who was chairman of the Judiciary Committee, advocated criminal penalties for CEOs and other executives, managers, and scientists in industries that knowingly manufactured and sold products for which there was clear evidence of adverse public health or environmental impact. However, Congress wasn't ready for the concept that people who went to church and came from Yale or Harvard could possibly be criminals. The legislation did not get a warm reception on Capitol Hill.

Today, I believe the time has come for a public health crimes tribunal, like the war crimes tribunal. Bulletproof documentation exists detailing acts of manipulation, suppression, distortion, and destruction of data by a wide range of corporations, resulting in disease and death.

What can we conclude from all of this? We know how to avoid the majority of cancers. From the point of view of self-interest, it's important for everybody to have this information and to spread it nationally. It's also incumbent on us to draw attention to the adverse impacts of runaway technologies and to get citizens nationwide concerned about them, using cancer as the most powerful paradigm, symbol, and metaphor of their dangers, and a metaphor for failed public policy. All this must be clearly recognized if we are to win the losing war against cancer.

Hoxsey: When Healing
Becomes a Crime

Kenny Ausubel

THERE IS ANOTHER CANCER WAR—against "unproven" alternative cancer therapies. But is the medical standard of proof a double standard?

In February 2001, a federal government—sponsored report published under the auspices of the National Institutes of Health (NIH) reported finding "noteworthy cases of survival" among cancer patients using the Hoxsey herbal treatment. After seventy-five years, Uncle Sam was finally giving a state nod to what is arguably the most notorious alternative cancer therapy in American history.

In the 1950s, at the height of organized medicine's crusade against the Hoxsey Cancer Clinics, the American Medical Association crystallized the medical establishment's sentiments in its supremely influential *Journal of the American Medical Association (JAMA)*. "It is fair to observe that the American Medical Association or any other association or individual has no need to go beyond the Hoxsey label to be convinced. Any such person who would seriously contend that scientific medicine is under any obligation to investigate such a mixture or its promoter is either stupid or dishonest."

The recent NIH report marks a surprising reversal in the long-standing medical civil war between conventional and alternative approaches. After a long exile, alternative therapies are now ascendant, riding a crest of popular demand, scientific validation, and commercial promise. The face of cancer treatment may soon become almost unrecognizable as valuable alternative therapies begin to permeate mainstream practice.

If Harry Hoxsey had lived to witness this apparent sea change in medicine, he might likely feel very mixed emotions. He would heartily cheer the grassroots surge propelling the movement, the same kind that once carried his Hoxsey Cancer Clinics to unmatched heights of popularity and validation. He would be exhilarated by the philosophical conversion of his enemies. But he would also be cynical, suspicious that a clinging monopoly was fighting to save face and above all keep its corner of the cancer market. But then, Hoxsey survived decades of being "hunted like a wild beast" only to see his clinics padlocked without the scientific test he relentlessly sought. He died a broken man, anguished over the future he felt humanity had been robbed of. Yet the Hoxsey treatment did live on, thriving as an underground legend, attracting more patients today than any of the other banished therapies, irrepressible after all.

The astonishing saga of the rise and fall and rebirth of Hoxsey provides a classic case history of the corrosive medical politics that have long prevented the fair investigation of promising alternative cancer therapies. Paradoxically, this long-standing denunciation has not been based on the objective scientific evidence that is supposed to determine the acceptance or rejection of medical therapies. Rather, the dismissal typifies the kind of pre-factual conclusion that has characterized "scientific" medicine's century-long pattern of condemnation without investigation.

In fact, the unspoken reason for the renaissance of alternative cancer therapies is sadly obvious: The medical establishment has largely lost its celebrated war on cancer, which is based on surgery, radiation, and chemotherapy. But what has remained hidden from most people is the existence of the other cancer war: organized medicine's zealous campaign against "unorthodox" cancer treatments and their practitioners. Over the course of the twentieth century, innovators such as Harry Hoxsey advanced more than one hundred alternative approaches, at least several of which have seemed to hold significant promise. Yet rather than being the subject of interest and investigation by mainstream medicine, their champions have been ridiculed, threatened with the loss of professional licenses, harassed, prosecuted, and driven out of the country.

The facts clearly reveal that these treatments have consistently been condemned, without investigation, by a consortium of interests: the American

Medical Association (AMA), the Food and Drug Administration (FDA), the National Cancer Institute (NCI), and the American Cancer Society (ACS), as well as certain large corporations that profit from the cancer industry. It is important to emphasize that this confederation of interests known as organized medicine consists principally of medical politicians and business interests, not practicing doctors. Physicians themselves have often objected to the unscientific rejection of alternative therapies and to restrictions on their own freedom to research or administer them.

The news blackout and disinformation campaign muffling this scandal have been so effective that most people do not happen into the underground of "disappeared" therapies until the fateful moment when they or their friends or relations are diagnosed with the dread disease. Usually only when fighting for their lives do patients discover the plethora of alternative cancer therapies claiming to offer hope and benefit, though with little if any scientific evidence to support the assertions. The story of Hoxsey sheds disturbing light on the many anecdotes of "people who got well when they weren't supposed to," as cancer surgeon Dr. Bernie Siegel terms these remarkable remissions in the netherworld of alternative therapies.

In 1840, Illinois horse farmer John Hoxsey found that his prize stallion had a malignant tumor on its right hock. As a Quaker, he couldn't bear to shoot the animal, so he put it out to pasture to die. Three weeks later, he noticed the tumor had stabilized, and he observed the animal browsing knee-deep in a corner of the pasture that contained a profusion of weeds, eating plants not part of its normal diet.

Within three months the tumor dried up and began to separate from the healthy tissue. The farmer retreated to the barn, where he began to experiment with these herbs revealed to him by "horse sense." He devised three formulas: an internal tonic, an herbal-mineral red paste, and a mineral-based yellow powder for external use. Within a year the horse was well and the veterinarian farmer became locally famous for treating animals with cancer.

The farmer's grandson, John C. Hoxsey, a veterinarian in southern Illinois, was the first to try the remedies on people, and he claimed positive results. His son Harry showed an early interest in the remedies and began working with him at the age of eight. John suffered an untimely accident when Harry was just fifteen. On his deathbed, John bequeathed the formulas to the boy with a charge to treat poor people for free and to minister to all races, creeds, and religions without prejudice. He asked that the treatment carry the Hoxsey name. Finally, he warned the boy that the "High Priests of Medicine" would fight him tooth and nail because he was taking money out of their pockets.

Harry Hoxsey worked in the coal mines, sold insurance, and pitched minor-league baseball for money, all the while planning to go to medical school to bring the treatment to the world, but soon found he had been blackballed after secretly treating several terminal patients who pled for their lives. With a local banker backing him, he founded the first Hoxsey Cancer Clinic in 1924, which was championed by the Taylorville, Illinois, chamber of commerce and opened to high school bands marching down Main Street.

As early word of his reputed successes spread, Hoxsey was invited to nearby Chicago, headquarters of the newly powerful AMA, to demonstrate the treatment. Grisly and indisputable photographic proof of the terminal case Hoxsey treated verifies that the patient recovered, living on for twelve years, cancer free.

Hoxsey then claimed that a high AMA official offered him a contract for the rights to the formulas. The alleged agreement assigned the property rights to a consortium of doctors including Dr. Morris Fishbein, the AMA chief and editor of *JAMA*. Hoxsey himself would be required to cease any further practice and would be awarded a small percentage of profits after ten years if the treatment panned out. When he invoked his Quaker father's deathbed charge that poor people be treated for free and that the treatment carry the family name, Hoxsey said the official threatened to hound him out of business unless he acquiesced.

Whatever may have happened, that's when the battle started. The AMA first denied the entire incident, then later acknowledged Hoxsey's patient's remission, though it credited it to prior treatments by surgery and radiation.

One thing was certain: Harry Hoxsey had made a very powerful enemy. By crossing swords with Fishbein, he alienated the most powerful figure in medicine. The AMA promptly dubbed him the worst cancer quack of the century, and he would be arrested more times than any other person in medical history.

Hoxsey quickly found himself opposing Fishbein's emerging medical-corporate complex. As late as 1900, medicine was therapeutically pluralistic and financially unprofitable. Doctors had the highest suicide rate of any profession, owing to their extreme poverty and low social standing. Fishbein's AMA would engineer an industrialized medical monoculture. What radically tipped the balance of power was an arranged marriage between big business and organized medicine. Under Fishbein's direction, the AMA sailed into a golden harbor of prosperity fueled by surgery, radiation, drugs, and a sprawling high-tech hospital system. The corporatization of medicine throttled diversity. The code word for competition was quackery.

It was easy for the medical profession to paint Hoxsey as a quack: He fit the image perfectly. Brandishing his famed tonic bottle, the ex — coal miner arrived straight from central casting, the very stereotype of the snake-oil salesman. When the AMA coerced the pathologist who performed Hoxsey's biopsies to cease and desist, Hoxsey could no longer verify his reputed successes. Organized medicine quickly adopted the stance that his alleged cures fell into three categories: those who never had cancer in the first place; those who were cured by prior radiation and surgery; and those who died. In exasperation, Hoxsey attempted an end run, approaching the National Cancer Institute. In close collaboration with the AMA, the federal agency refused his application for a test of the remedies because the medical records he supplied did not include the results of all the biopsies performed on his patients, biopsies doctors refused to give him.

Meanwhile, Hoxsey struck oil in Texas and used his riches to promote his burgeoning clinic and finance his court battles. Piqued by Hoxsey's rise, Fishbein struck back in the public media, penning an inflammatory article in the Hearst Sunday papers entitled "Blood Money," a classic example of purple prose and yellow journalism. Outraged, Hoxsey sued Fishbein. In two consecutive trials, Hoxsey beat Fishbein, becoming the first person labeled a quack to defeat the AMA in court. During the trials, Hoxsey's lawyers revealed that

Fishbein had failed anatomy in medical school, never completed his internship, and never practiced a day of medicine in his entire career.

By now Fishbein was mired in multiple scandals, including his effective but unpopular obstruction of national health insurance at a time when doctors had become the richest professionals in the country and *JAMA* the most profitable publication in the world. Drug ads powered *JAMA*, but its biggest single advertiser in the 1940s was Phillip Morris. (Camel had the largest booth at the AMA's 1948 convention, boasting in its ads that "more doctors smoke Camels than any other cigarette.") Enmeshed in controversy, Fishbein's stock was trading low, and, shortly after his first loss to Hoxsey, the AMA chief was deposed in a humiliating spectacle.

Ironically, Hoxsey's stunning dark-horse victory against the "most terrifying trade organization on Earth" only ended up precipitating heightened repression. He immediately faced a decade-long "quackdown" by the FDA.

By the 1950s, Hoxsey was riding the wave of what was arguably the largest alternative medicine movement in American history. A survey by the Chicago Medical Society showed 85 percent of people still using "drugless healers." Hoxsey's Dallas stronghold grew to be the world's largest privately owned cancer center, with 12,000 patients and branches in seventeen states. Congressmen, judges, and even some doctors ardently supported his quest for a scientific investigation. Two federal courts upheld the therapeutic value of the treatment. Even his archenemies, the AMA and the FDA, admitted that the therapy did cure certain forms of cancer. *JAMA* itself had published the research of a respected physician who got results superior to surgery by using a red paste identical to Hoxsey's for skin cancers, including lethal melanoma, a skin cancer that also spreads internally.

Medical authorities escalated their quackdown in the McCarthyite wake of the late 1950s. On the heels of a California law criminalizing all cancer treatments except surgery, radiation, and chemotherapy, in 1960 the federal government finally outlawed Hoxsey entirely in the United States on questionable technicalities. Chief nurse Mildred Nelson moved the clinic to Tijuana in 1963, abandoning any hope of operating in the United States. It was the

first alternative clinic to set up shop south of the border. Mildred quietly treated
another 30,000 patients there until her death in 1999. Like Hoxsey, she claimed
a high success rate, but her contention is unverified since the treatment has
yet to be rigorously tested.

Hoxsey never claimed to have a panacea or cure-all. He maintained that
Dallas doctors used his clinic as a dumping ground for hopeless cases and that
the great majority of patients he got were terminal, having already had the limit
of surgery and radiation. Hoxsey said he cured about 25 percent of those. With
virgin cases with no prior treatment, he claimed an 80 percent success rate.
Seventy-five years after Hoxsey began, why do we still not know the validity of this claims?

Organized medicine has systematically dismissed alternative cancer therapies as "unproven" and lacking the rigorous scientific proof of clinical trials.
But if the Hoxsey treatment is unproven, it's not disproven. Like virtually all
the "unorthodox" cancer therapies over the course of the twentieth century,
it was politically railroaded rather than medically tested. However, over the
last few decades, controlled laboratory tests have shown all the individual
herbs in the internal tonic to possess anti-tumor and anti-cancer properties, as
I documented in detail in my book on Hoxsey, *When Healing Becomes a Crime.*
Though the formula has never been tested as a whole entity, clearly there is a
credible scientific basis for looking at it. Organized medicine has not disputed
the effectiveness of the external remedies since 1950, and the red paste (Mohs
treatment) is listed in *Taber's Medical Encyclopedia* as a "standard treatment,"
though it is seldom used.

After all, plants are the cornerstone of pharmaceutical drugs. The very
word "drug" derives from the Dutch term *droog,* which means "to dry," since
people have historically dried plants to make medicinal preparations. It is well
proven that many botanicals possess powerful anti-cancer properties. Numerous primary pharmaceuticals derive from plants, as do several major
chemotherapy drugs, such as Taxol, from the Pacific Yew tree, Vincristine and
Vinblastine, from the Madagascar periwinkle, and Camptothecin, from the
wood and bark of a Chinese tree. About 30 percent of chemotherapy drugs
altogether are derived from natural substances, mainly plants. A quarter of

modern drugs still contain a plant substance, and about half are modeled on plant chemistry.

During Hoxsey's era, surgery and radiation were primitive and excessive. Both were solely local treatments, reflecting the profession's belief that cancer was a local disease. As such, they could address just a quarter of all cases, claiming to cure only about a quarter of those. With the advent of toxic chemotherapy drugs in the 1950s, organized medicine at last acknowledged cancer as a systemic disease, which Hoxsey and the other "unorthodox" practitioners had been asserting all along.

Clearly, conventional cancer treatments have an important place in medicine and save lives. But since the 1950s, evidence has steadily accumulated that surgery, radiation, and chemotherapy are far less effective than the public is being led to believe. Investigative journalist Daniel Greenberg, writing in the *Columbia Journalism Review* in 1975, produced the first widely reported exposé showing that cancer survival rates had not progressed since the 1950s, and that improvements made from 1930 to 1950 were mainly a consequence of improved hospital nursing care and support systems. Greenberg found that even the valid improvements were very, very small, and that there had been no significant advancements in treating any of the major forms of cancer.

In 1969, Dr. Hardin Jones released a shocking report on this issue at the Science Writers Convention sponsored by the ACS. Jones, a respected professor of medical physics from the University of California at Berkeley and an expert on statistics and the effects of radiation and drugs, concluded that "the common malignancies show a remarkably similar rate of demise, whether treated or untreated." Joining the fray, Nobel laureate James Watson charged that the American public had been sold a "nasty bill of goods about cancer." This eminent codiscoverer of the DNA double helix remarked bluntly that the war on cancer was "a bunch of shit."

These "proven" cancer treatments are themselves largely unproven. The standard of proof for therapeutic efficacy is in fact a double standard. Surgery was grandfathered in as standard practice early in the twentieth century without randomized, double-blind clinical trials, which only became widespread in the 1960s, with the advent of chemotherapy. Its dangers and limitations have since been only superficially acknowledged or studied, and little is known about its efficacy in relation to a baseline marker of no treatment.

Like surgery, radiation therapy was grandfathered in without rigorous test-ing. Radiation is carcinogenic and mutagenic. In the few tests comparing ra-diation treatment against no treatment, according to Jones, "Most of the time, it makes not the slightest difference if the machine is turned on or not." Jones went even further, saying, "My studies have proved conclusively that un-treated cancer victims actually live up to four times longer." Radiation is often combined with surgery despite the fact that tests have generally shown it made no apparent favorable difference. A recent study with patients with the most common form of lung cancer found that postoperative radiation therapy, which is routinely given, actually raises the relative risk of death by 21 percent, and is most detrimental to those in the early stages of illness. Nevertheless, radia-tion is used on about half of cancer patients.

It was into this disappointing setting that chemotherapy entered as the next great hope of cancer treatment. Chemotherapy drugs are poisons that are in-discriminate killers of cells, both healthy and malignant. The strategy is quite literally to kill the cancer without killing the patient. By the mid-1980s, promi-nent members of medical orthodoxy had published unsettling assessments that could no longer be dismissed. Writing in *Scientific American*, Dr. John Cairns, who was then at Harvard Medical School, found that chemotherapy was able to save the lives of just 2 to 3 percent of cancer patients, usually those with the rarest kinds of the disease. By medicine's own standards, at best, chemother-apy is unproven against 90 percent of adult solid tumors, the huge majority of common cancers resulting in death. Moreover, true placebo controls have been almost abandoned in the testing of chemotherapy. Drug regimen is tested against drug regimen, and doctors hardly ever look at whether the drugs do better than simple good nursing care. Because chemotherapy drugs are out-right poisons, many carcinogenic, the drugs themselves can cause "treatment deaths" and additional cancers. One study showed that among women sur-viving ovarian cancer, those who had been given chemotherapy developed leukemia at a rate one hundred times that of women who had not received chemotherapy. In some studies, when chemotherapy and radiation were combined, the incidence of secondary tumors was about twenty-five times the expected rate. Nevertheless, chemotherapy is given to 80 percent of patients.

Amazingly, 85 percent of prescribed standard medical treatments lack scientific validation, according to the *New York Times*. Richard Smith, editor of the *British Medical Journal*, suggests that "this is partly because only one percent of the articles in medical journals are scientifically sound, and partly because many treatments have never been assessed at all."

A hundred years from now, medicine will likely come to regard some of these "proven" cancer treatments the way we now remember the use of mercury and bloodletting. As Dr. Abigail Zuger wrote in the *New York Times*, contemplating the hundredth anniversary of the 1899 *Merck Manual:* "We have harnessed our own set of poisons for medical treatment; in a hundred years a discussion of cancer chemotherapy may read as chillingly as endorsements of strychnine for tuberculosis and arsenic for diabetes do today."

The civil war between Hoxsey and organized medicine has largely reflected a trade war. Profitability has often been the driving force behind the adoption of official therapeutics. At over $110 billion a year just in the United States, cancer is big business, a whopping 10 percent of the national health care bill. The typical cancer patient spends upward of $100,000 on treatment. It is estimated that each hospital admission for cancer produces two to three times the billings of a typical non-cancer admission. More people work in the field than die from the disease each year. According to Dr. Samuel Epstein, "For decades, the war on cancer has been dominated by powerful groups of interlocking professional and financial interests, with the highly profitable drug development system at its hub." Global sales of chemotherapy drugs in 1997 were $30.9 billion, about $12 billion of it in the United States.

Pharmaceutical companies pin the high costs of drugs on the forbidding expense of testing and approving each new drug, now pegged at $500 million. In fact, this prohibitive figure has served as a barrier to entry for all but giant corporations. The entire system is founded on patents, twenty-year exclusive licenses that provide monopoly protection. As an herbal product, the Hoxsey tonic cannot be patented and therefore occupies the status of an orphan drug that no company will develop. While it has approved about forty highly toxic cancer drugs, the FDA has yet to approve a single nontoxic cancer agent or one not patented by a major pharmaceutical company.

Alternative therapies are finally emerging in part because of the dramatic cost savings they represent, and because at least some may well represent a major new profit center. "Alternative medicine is clearly the largest growth industry in health care today," wrote Jane Brody in the *New York Times* in 1998. Dr. David Eisenberg of Harvard Medical School surveyed the American public and found that 42 percent were using alternative therapies in 1997. The number of visits to alternative practitioners exceeded total visits to primary care physicians. Spending was conservatively estimated at $21.2 billion, with at least $12.2 billion paid out-of-pocket by committed customers. Total out-of-pocket expenditures for alternative therapies were comparable with expenditures for all physician services.

The numbers are no less dramatic for cancer treatment. A national study estimated 64 percent of cancer patients to be using alternative therapies. A recent survey at M. D. Anderson Cancer Center, the world's largest, with 13,000 patients, found an astounding 83 percent using alternatives. Major corporations are already entering the alternative marketplace. Procter & Gamble initially spent millions sponsoring the research of Dr. Nick Gonzalez, who took up the work of Donald Kelley, a dentist who reputedly cured himself of terminal pancreatic cancer using enzymes and other nutritional means. Nestlé has also financed the work of Dr. Gonzalez. A pilot study of pancreatic cancer patients treated with enzymes provided better results than had been seen in the history of medicine for a disease that is 95 percent incurable. The subjects lived an average of triple the usual survival time, and two patients have lived for four and five years with no detectable disease. These studies led to a $1.4 million grant to Columbia University College of Physicians and Surgeons by the NIH's National Center for Complementary and Alternative Medicine (NCCAM), supervised by the NCI. The engagement of large corporations catapulted a formerly reviled treatment to instant plausibility. When big companies start to take a stake in alternative cancer therapies, it signifies the maturation of a market and consecrates a political realignment.

Both M. D. Anderson and Memorial Sloan-Kettering Cancer Center have been testing green tea, or more accurately several of its active ingredients, for anti-cancer properties. Because various studies have shown that green tea reduces the risk of colorectal, lung, esophageal, and pancreatic cancers, the Lipton tea company is also testing the substance at the University of Arizona.

In association with the NCI, M. D. Anderson is set to evaluate shark cartilage, which is reputed to have anti-cancer activity and is widely used by a cancer underground in the United States and abroad. (Sadly, this market surge is further endangering several shark species.) The University of Toronto is testing mistletoe, a folk remedy for cancer espoused by the Austrian spiritual philosopher Rudolf Steiner, the originator of Waldorf education and Biodynamic farming. Mistletoe has shown anti-tumor effects in both human and animal studies in Germany.

The release of the report on Hoxsey through the NIH's NCCAM is a harbinger of the changes to come. As the report concludes, further investigation "is justified not only because of the public health issue to justify the large number of patients who seek treatment at this clinic, but also because of the several noteworthy cases of survival." The report specifically notes a seven-year survivor of melanoma who had no treatment besides Hoxsey's tonic and external salves. Average survival time for advanced melanoma is seven months. If such a remarkable remission occurred using conventional treatments, it would be front-page news worldwide.

"It's interesting to contemplate the dilemma that the National Cancer Institute is in," conjectures Ralph Moss, an adviser to the NCCAM and NCI and a respected researcher and author on both alternative and conventional cancer treatments:

> If they do decide to do the tests, then there's always that possibility— and I think it's a damn good possibility—that some of these treatments are going to turn out to be quite valuable. If they decide not to do the tests, there's going to be tremendous fury in Congress and the public, because what then are they about? If they're not about scientific testing, what good are they? Why are we wasting our money?
>
> What we're saying is: Prove them or disprove them. We've had

seventy-five years of Hoxsey. Does it work? Doesn't it work? Nobody knows. How do you know? Short of good studies, how does
one decide issues like that? We don't want people doing something
if it's not going to work for them, not in terms of just conventional
treatment, but alternative treatments as well.

The best-case scenario is that some tests will be carried out with
the imprimatur of NCI, NCCAM, and probably other collaborative
centers like the University of Texas and Columbia. Some of those will
show that there's no effectiveness, and some of them will probably
show that there is effectiveness in some treatments. The ones that are
shown to be effective that are funded by and based on NCI-reported
research are then going to be published in major medical journals. The
first one that validates a nontoxic treatment is the beginning of the
end of this Middle Ages that we're in. Because once one goes through
the door, then a lot of others are going through the door, and that's
what they're afraid of. They're afraid that, if a Hoxsey were proven
to be effective, the public will run to it because nobody wants the
chemo drugs. If chemo is the only choice, then they'll reluctantly take
it, but the minute it's known there is something nontoxic out there,
everybody's going to want it.

The abiding truth for cancer patients is that they want unrestricted access
to all treatments. According to one analysis, only about 5 percent entirely aban-
don conventional cancer care even when pursuing an alternative. What patients seek is the best of all worlds, an expanded menu of options supported
by access to credible information. The stereotype that orthodoxy has long put
forth of poor, credulous cancer patients ripe for exploitation by clever pro-
moters turns out to be false. In a study by sociologist Barrie Cassileth, the profile
of patients using alternative cancer therapies describes well-educated, middle-
income, often female clients who have done a considerable amount of due dili-
gence before making their choice.

While physicians fought fiercely for their professional sovereignty during the twentieth century, the greater social issue today is the sovereignty of

the patient. In a market economy, goes the old saw, the customer is always right. The AMA's Oliver Field, an architect of the aggressive repression against Hoxsey and myriad other "quack" therapies in the 1950s, responded surprisingly when I posed to him the polarizing question of freedom of medical choice: "This is a free country. You pays your money and you takes your choice. If it's wrong, you're the one who's going to suffer."

It was anomalous to hear the former head of the AMA's Bureau of Investigation, which once boasted a list of over 300,000 "quacks," echo the words of his past nemesis. Judge William Hawley Atwell, who ruled twice in Hoxsey's favor in federal courts and fully affirmed the therapy's value, had stated in 1949 regarding Hoxsey's victory over Dr. Morris Fishbein, "So I wish to say, pay your money and take your choice. Those who need a doctor, if you think one side is the best, go and get him. If you think the other side is best, you certainly have the right to go and get him. This is a free country; that is what we stand for in America."

Why was the Hoxsey therapy not investigated in the first place seventy-five years ago? The overarching truth is that it has been politically railroaded instead of medically tested. The medical civil war has distorted cancer from a medical question into a political issue. The many practitioners and doctors thrust involuntarily into the front lines of the cancer wars would surely prefer to settle the question in a clinic or laboratory rather than a courtroom. Meanwhile, cancer patients remain trapped in the crossfire, fighting for their lives.

Part IV

Nature, Culture, and Medicine

Healing, Nature,
and Modern Medicine

Andrew Weil

Dr. Andrew Weil is perhaps the Dr. Spock of the next generation of physicians. That's Dr. Benjamin Spock, not the Spock of Star Trek, *though Andy has certainly gone where no doctor has gone before. His brilliance is matched by his courage as a physician-diplomat willing to challenge a profession often being dragged kicking and screaming into the twenty-first century. He has taken on the daunting task of re-fashioning a system that is in many ways in crisis.*

Sometimes people mistake his stance as exclusively favoring natural medicine. In fact, he is equally committed to conventional allopathic medicine, which has much to recommend it. But he is willing to explore everything and to use whatever really works. Above all, he treats people, not diseases.

He may be one of very few doctors in the country who were botany majors in college. After graduating from Harvard Medical School in the 1960s, he worked for thirteen years on the research staff of the Harvard Botanical Museum and trav-eled the world to study ancient healing and medical lineages, from Ayurveda to shamanism. He has been relentlessly attacked by forces within the medical profession who discount alternative therapies as "unproven." The irony is that according to med-icine's own standards, 85 percent of prescribed standard medical treatments lack sci-entific validation.

Andy has played a central role in bringing about the historic transition to an in-tegrative medicine. He is best known for his prodigious output of eloquent popular books and lectures. He has written a fistful of classics such as Natural Health, Natural Med-icine, The Natural Mind, Spontaneous Healing, *and, most recently, the popular best-sellers* Eight Weeks to Optimum Health *and* Eating Well for Optimum Health. *He also publishes a newsletter and website rich with practical information.*

But in many ways his most important work takes place in the trenches of medical education. He is director of the Program in Integrative Medicine at the College of Medicine at the University of Arizona, a visionary pilot effort to include alternative therapies in the training of physicians. He has helped create a consortium of sixteen Academic Health Centers for Integrative Medicine. He is working to change the entire culture of medicine. And in addition to all of that, he manages to maintain his general practice in Tucson.

Above all, Andy's mission has been about reconnecting medicine with nature, and he stands as one of the most brilliant and heartfelt advocates for the ecological health of the planet. It's no coincidence that he's also a passionate gardener and cook. As Erma Bombeck said, "Never go to a doctor whose office plants have died!" Andy's plants are thriving.

❦   ❦   ❦

I'M A PHYSICIAN IN TUCSON, ARIZONA, where I practice what I call natural and preventive medicine. Really I think I just practice common-sense medicine, but it's not what most doctors do. As a result of my botanical training, a lot of the prescribing that I do is botanical. During my freshman year at Harvard in 1960, I had no idea what I wanted to do in life (I still really don't). Thumbing through the course catalogue, I thought I would take one of everything and I found a course called "Plants and Human Affairs." What a wonderful name for a college course! It was about the relationships that human beings form with plants.

It turned out, although I didn't know it then, that it was the oldest course given continuously at Harvard. At the time that I took it, the senior lecturer was Paul Mangelsdorf, who had done a great deal of work on the ancestry of corn, but the main lecturer was Richard Evans Schultes, who later became head of the Harvard Botanical Museum. You had to go over the museum to sign up for this course. It was an old, gloomy Victorian brick building, and when I went over there, in the fall of 1960, out of the entrance came a being I had never seen the likes of before. It was a proto-hippie—a long-haired man who I'm sure had been up in the Library of Economic Botany, which had the greatest collection in the country of books on psychoactive plants.

I got the immediate sense that this was someplace I wanted be. You had to climb up stair after stair, past exhibits of South American blowguns and an exhibit on ayahuasca. Every week we had a lab. There was a Deepfreeze in this course, with tropical fruits from all over the world, and we had a fruit-of-the-week to try every week. In the first lab we made a typical Mexican meal. Schultes had a Mexican graduate student then, and his wife would come in to lead this exercise. We had subsequent laboratories on making ink and soap and perfume. We made whiskey out of corn. We had a drug lab in which we tried exotic Amazonian drugs. This was 1960, remember. Later I became a laboratory instructor in the course.

I think this was the only college course in which I learned practical things. It was real stuff, some of which I still use. Anyway, I have an undergraduate degree in botany. Actually, it's in "biology" because there wasn't a botany department at Harvard. Botany was a unit of the biology department and it was seen as a very old-fashioned, musty sort of biology. There was constant rumbling by the molecular biologists to push it out into a farther and farther corner of the university. I am sorry to tell you that in the years since then, I have met only two other physicians who were botany majors as undergraduates, and neither of them uses his botanical training in his medical practice.

At all the meetings that I go to in which I hear people talking about plant chemistry, medicinal plants, herbal medicine, the FDA, and politics, there are never any practicing physicians. It's botanists, plant chemists, and people working in pharmaceutical laboratories; almost never do practitioners of medicine have a working knowledge of botany. There are many people out there who have great knowledge of plants and their structure and chemistry but who have no knowledge of real-world medicine.

And there are people who deal with patients who have not the slightest interest in or knowledge of botany. I think that's sad. I feel lonely in my position, and sad because it shows the degree to which science and medicine have separated themselves from nature and separated us from nature. Two hundred years ago, if you wanted to study medicine, you had to know botany because most of medicine consisted of giving people preparations of plants. Even today, many of the drugs in clinical use are of plant origin or are molecular variations of chemicals originally discovered in plants.

Yet to most doctors today, the idea of giving a patient a plant seems at best hopelessly old-fashioned, and at worst outright dangerous and unscientific. There's almost no dialogue between the fields of medicine and botany. Pharmacy maintained a better connection with its botanical origins, but every pharmacy college in the country has dropped pharmacognosy as a required course. Pharmacognosy was the branch of pharmacy that dealt with the discovery, extraction, and identification of new drugs from natural sources. It was the living heart of pharmacy and that field's connection to nature.

Today, I'm sorry to say—and I don't mean this with disrespect—it seems to me that the only requirements you really need to be a pharmacist are not to be color blind and to be able to read and count. All the good stuff that used to go on, like the compounding of natural remedies, is gone.

The separation between medicine and botany has enormous consequences for our society, because fundamentally, healing is a natural process. If you want to understand healing and how to make people better, you must understand the ways of nature. You should live close to nature and develop a feel for natural processes. Not only does medical training today isolate people from nature, but our medicine and our science even contribute to a fear of nature.

As an example: Most people in this country think that if they randomly eat plants in the backyard, the likelihood is that they'll die. Actually, the percentage of plants that can kill you is very, very small. The percentage of plants that can do wonderful things for you is probably also relatively small. And the vast majority probably aren't going to affect you one way or the other. But most people have that fear, and that fear is very much reinforced by medical scientists. I have a colleague in the College of Pharmacy at the University of Arizona, where I teach, who periodically writes popular articles about the dangers of herbal teas. He tells people that if you are enough of a consumer of health food store products, sooner or later you're going to be poisoned.

There are a few herbs to be concerned about, but most of the products that you find in health food stores are not dangerous and certainly not deadly. There are many questions about whether herbal products are efficacious, whether they're overpriced, and whether false claims are made for them, but not about whether they're going to do you in. The message that's not overtly stated but is between the lines is that nature is fundamentally wild, dangerous, and unpredictable. It's out to get you, whereas the products of pharmaceutical laboratories are safe. That message is especially annoying because it's actually the other way around, and I say that as a doctor who often has to deal with the casualties of pharmaceutical science. I see many patients who have been seriously hurt by taking pharmaceutical drugs. In fact, the single greatest black mark against conventional medicine is the amount of toxicity that it causes as a result of its preference for chemical drugs that are very strong and very fast acting.

The whole emphasis in medicine has been to discover bioactive compounds that produce ever more dramatic effects ever more quickly. It's sometimes useful to have such compounds at your disposal. In an emergency, where there's a real crisis and you don't have time, it's nice to have a drug that's going to work within minutes and produce an immediate effect. But such conditions amount to a very small percentage of total illness. Nevertheless, most regular medicine is geared toward treating all illness as if it were a crisis. Conventional medicine is good at the management of crises, but it deals with *everything* in that mode. It brings out the heavy artillery, the big guns, for everything. There's a huge price to pay for reliance on pharmaceutical agents of that sort, and that price is toxicity.

Any dedicated patient sooner or later is going to experience an adverse drug reaction. That's a certainty, I guarantee you. Adverse drug reactions can be as mild as hives and as major as death and permanent disability. This is a huge problem in our medicine and in our society today.

Because Chinese medicine, like many older medical traditions, is based on conceptions of health and illness very different from those of Western medicine, it is an interesting example to consider. Chinese medicine is mostly concerned with energy and energy flows through the body. In the Chinese conception, all illness results from imbalances of energy in the body. Chinese diagnosis tries to determine where those imbalances are in the body and whether they are excesses or deficiencies of energy. Chinese treatment aims to correct the balances, bringing more energy to places that are deficient and draining energy away from places that have too much of it.

Chinese medicine places much more emphasis on prevention than does Western medicine. We have a specialty called preventive medicine, but it's not what I consider the real thing. Preventive medicine as it's now set up is concerned mostly with immunization and public sanitation. Those are important, but they're not the essence. Preventive medicine should be about teaching people how to change their lives in order to reduce risks of disease. It should be about how to design optimal diets so that we don't fall prey to the diseases that kill and disable people prematurely. It should be about teaching people to handle stress in ways that protect their bodies, and teaching people how to breathe properly so that their nervous systems are nurtured. None of that is now taught in preventive medicine training.

In Chinese medicine there is an idea I find very powerful. It's that there are two categories of illness—visible and invisible—and that visible illness is always preceded by invisible illness. What Chinese doctors mean by invisible illness is a disturbance in the energy dynamics of the body, in the energy flow pattern. They say that if that's not corrected, sooner or later it will crystallize into a disturbance of the structure of the body, and that at that point it is no longer so easy to change. Once disease has become fixed in the structure of the body, it takes much more energy, time, and effort to correct it, and the chance of correcting it is less.

If you try to talk about that concept with Western doctors, if they listen to you at all, they'll shake their heads in disbelief. It doesn't compute. For one thing, it's very difficult to talk about energy with Western doctors and scientists, even though energy is a hard, physical concept. In physics, energy is defined as the ability to do work. Yet when you talk about energy in a biological sense, it becomes a kind of buzzword like "natural" that types you as New Age and mystical, meaning not scientific, and people stop listening.

The Chinese concept of invisible illness, like Chinese medical science in general, developed in an absence of familiarity with the detailed inner structure of the human body. Instead, it is a science that concerns function and functional relationships in the human body. Where Chinese doctors diagnose a disturbance in a body function in the invisible stage, we in the West often use the term "functional illness," meaning an illness in which there is a disturbance of function but nothing materially, structurally wrong. Let's say a patient comes in complaining of urinary incontinence, and you do all the tests, and they all come out normal. The Western doctor says, "This is a functional urinary disturbance." True. But the connotation in Western medicine of the word "functional" is "unreal." When we diagnose a patient as having a functional complaint, we mean it's all in the patient's head, and therefore we don't have to bother with it.

In Chinese medicine the problem would be taken more seriously because it's at this stage that you can it with the least effort. The fact that Western medicine relegates the whole category of functional illness to the status of "unreal" is an indication of the materialism of Western science and medicine. What is real in materialistic science is that which you can touch and measure. If you can't measure it or find a structural correlate, then it's not real.

In Chinese medicine, many treatments are used: adjustment of diet, massage, acupuncture (a completely unique treatment that doesn't occur anywhere else in the world), and a great deal of prescribing of remedies, the vast majority of which are herbal. The Chinese herbal pharmacopoeia is vast. It would be the work of many lifetimes to make sense of it. It's rivaled only by the Indian pharmacopoeia, which is probably even richer because India is subtropical and tropical and has an even greater diversity of plants.

There are some interesting aspects of Chinese herbal medicine that are very different from Western herbal medicine. The Chinese insist that when you find a plant in nature that has an effect, there is no point in isolating elements of that plant. The Chinese are interested to know about the components of plants and what pharmacological actions you can expect of them, but they will only give the plants in whole form, as teas and extracts. They will not tamper with their chemistry.

In the West our approach is reductionistic. You find a plant in nature, and you want to identify the one compound in it that has the most interesting effects. Then you isolate that, purify it, make it available for medical use in pure form, and if possible, tinker with the molecule to step up the intensity of the effect even further. That's the road Western pharmaceutical science has gone down.

Some Western pharmaceutical companies now sense that there are a lot of potential hits in the Chinese herbal pharmacopoeia; some of them have been reported in Western scientific journals, such as the discovery of the anti-malarial activity of a plant called *Artemisia annua*, which grows in our country as well. Called Sweet Annie, it works against the malaria parasite by a different mechanism from any of the pharmaceutical drugs that we have, drugs to which many malaria organisms have now become resistant. In the light of these discoveries, a number of Western pharmaceutical companies have signed exclusive contracts with China to get the rights to a particular plant, but their intention is to isolate one chemical from it and eventually patent and market that chemical or a variant of it, violating the Chinese principle that plant remedies should be given in whole form.

The Chinese pharmacopoeia has a very interesting scheme of classifying drugs that runs totally contrary to our ideas. The Chinese posit three categories called superior drugs, middle drugs, and inferior drugs.

An inferior drug in Chinese medicine is one that has a specific effect on a specific disease. In Western medicine, that is the highest ideal of a drug: the magic bullet, a drug that has a precise effect on a precise condition. In fact, in Western medicine, if a drug begins to work in too many conditions, we lose interest in it, because we think that means it can't be working by a specific biochemical mechanism.

Superior drugs in Chinese medicine are the ones that work for everything. They're panaceas, cure-alls. The word "panacea" has dreadful associations in Western medicine. It's snake oil. One of the superior drugs in Chinese medicine is ginseng. The Latin name of ginseng is *Panax*, from the same root as "panacea," cure-all, because so many claims are made for its benefits. Because it was good for everything, Western scientists took no interest in it.

There are two species of ginseng. There's Asian ginseng, *Panax ginseng*, and there's American ginseng, a Native American species called *Panax quinquefolius*, native to the woods of eastern North America.

In the early 1500s, the first Westerners—Jesuit missionaries from Portugal—reached the imperial court at Peking. The Chinese emperor immediately realized the utility of Jesuits. Here was a worldwide network of intelligent people in communication with each other. The Chinese gave these early missionaries samples of ginseng because even at that time, demand for that herb far exceeded supply, and the price was astronomical. The Chinese were constantly searching for new sources because it was in such demand.

The Jesuits were asked to send samples of ginseng around to their missions to see if they could find it growing anywhere else in the world. Eventually, in the early 1600s, some of the samples reached a mission in eastern Quebec. Jesuits there noticed a plant growing in the woods that looked similar. This was American ginseng. As far as I can determine, there was little Native American use of this plant. Its medicinal activity was not much known in America.

The Canadian Jesuits sent samples of their ginseng to Peking, and eventually word came back, "Send as much as you can." So there began a trade in American ginseng to China that reached such proportions that within about fifty years, our native ginseng had been exterminated from the woods of eastern Canada. Harvesting then spread down into New York State and over to Ohio. A lot of the earlier settlers of the west made their living picking ginseng. Daniel Boone was a ginseng hunter, for example; that's how he made his living.

Throughout all these years, tonnage of ginseng was shipped to China, continuing up to our own times. No American scientist ever thought to study ginseng to see if there was anything in it that made it worthwhile. Through all this time, all Americans thought about it was that it was something funny that people on the other side of the ocean paid money for. Because ginseng was said to do so many things, it couldn't possibly be a real drug. That conception prevented plant scientists from even looking at the chemistry of ginseng to see if there was anything there that might have bioactivity. Research on ginseng in this part of the world has only been done in the past twenty to twenty-five years. It turns out that the root is loaded with bioactive compounds that work on the pituitary-adrenal axis, activity that can explain the actions attributed to it in China.

Many of the drugs in the superior category in the Chinese pharmacopoeia are mushrooms. There is an enormous difference in cultural attitudes toward mushrooms in Asia and the English-speaking world. Gordon Wasson, a New York banker who died in 1986, made his avocation the study of mushrooms, and rediscovered the psilocybin mushroom rituals of Mexico. He wrote a book called *Mushrooms, Russia and History* in which he argued that all human cultures can be divided into what he called mycophilic and mycophobic: mushroom-loving and mushroom-fearing or -hating.

The English-speaking world is at one extreme of the spectrum: mycophobia. That may not seem apparent; we put mushrooms on pizzas and steaks. But if you compare us with a truly mycophilic culture like the Chinese, Japanese, or some Slavic populations, you see the differences. In any grocery store that you go into in Japan you will find a dozen different species of cultivated mushrooms for sale. Until very recently we have cultivated only one species, the common *agaricus.*

In some Slavic languages there are dozens of words for mushrooms. In English we have only "mushroom," "toadstool," and "fungus." In these Slavic cultures people make centerpieces for their tables out of poisonous mushrooms that they consider beautiful. They take mushrooms to bed with them. They fondle them. They talk to them. They kiss them. You don't find people in Australia, Great Britain, Canada, and the United States acting that way.

One of the characteristics of Asian mycophilic cultures is their esteem for mushrooms as powerful medicines. In fact, they are highly represented in the category of superior drugs. In the West, we have never looked to mushrooms as sources of new drugs—a failure that comes entirely out of our cultural attitudes. The fact that Western pharmaceutical scientists have never looked to mushrooms as sources of new drugs is irrational. First, if you want to find new drugs, you look to areas of nature that have very diverse chemistry, and of all the productions of nature, mushrooms have some of the richest and strangest chemical diversity. They contain very unusual compounds that occur nowhere else, many with novel molecular structures.

Second, there's a lot of bioactivity in mushrooms. Many have chemicals that produce effects in animals. Finally, they have a lot of toxins in them, not just deadly ones but a whole range of lesser sorts of toxins. If you want to find new drugs, you look to poisons, because there's no difference between a drug and a poison except dose. The word "pharmacology" means the study of poisons.

"Toxicology" also has an interesting derivation. It comes from the Greek word for bow, as in bow and arrow, *taxos*. One writer commenting on that said, "Imagine how many poisoned arrows must have flown and found their mark before the word took on the connotation of poison." At any rate, pharmacology is the study of poisons. Many poisons become useful drugs if you can lower the dose enough. All drugs become poisons if you push the dose high enough.

Finally, the greatest single success of the modern pharmaceutical industry has been the isolation of antibiotics from very closely related organisms, what are called lower fungi (molds). Mushrooms are higher fungi. For all these reasons you would think that pharmaceutical scientists would have looked at mushrooms, especially since in the traditional pharmacopoeias of China and Japan mushrooms are so frequently represented as having superior effects, such as extending longevity and promoting resistance to stress of all kinds. But it hasn't been done.

Superior drugs in Chinese medicine are those that strengthen the defensive function of the human body. Ancient Chinese medical scientists did not know the immune system as we know it. Although they didn't know about tonsils, adenoids, the spleen, and lymph nodes, they had a clear concept of a defensive functional sphere of the human body. They thought that one profitable line of medical treatment was to find ways of strengthening that function. In the West, most of our effort at treatment has been to try to identify agents of disease and then to develop weapons against the agents, to oppose external agents of disease.

The emphasis in the East has been to strengthen internal resistance to whatever comes at you from outside. Obviously both of those approaches have their own validity and purpose, and it seems to me that the best kind of medicine would synthesize them; you try to do both. The way these superior drugs work in Chinese medicine is by strengthening internal resistance, so of course they're going to be good for everything. They're going to increase resistance to stress and help with viral diseases, infectious diseases, cancer, and allergy, because if you are more resistant and more balanced inside, then you can move through the world and not get knocked off balance so easily. That's a perfectly understandable explanation for how a drug could work in many different conditions.

One of the reasons that I feel compelled to do the work I do is that I believe medicine is a big piece of the logjam that keeps the world going in the destructive direction it has been going. One could make a convincing case, and some people have actually done it, that medicine in our culture serves the same function as religion in traditional societies. Medical doctors are the priests of technological society. People invest the same kind of belief in doctors that they do in shamans in shamanistic cultures.

In a shamanistic culture, if an event happens that's never happened before, like an eclipse of the sun, people go to the shaman to ask for an interpretation as to whether it is good or evil. In our society, if something new comes along, we go to medical scientists and ask if it is good or bad for our health. It's the same process. The problem is that medical doctors today are unable to serve the function of priests and shamans because of their limiting philosophy and belief system. The essential function of a priest or shaman is to serve as an intermediary between the visible world and the invisible world, between the world of matter and the world of spirit. If you don't believe in an invisible world, if you don't believe that there is anything other than matter, how can you possibly serve that function?

I see all sorts of patients. About 10 percent of the people who come to see me are well and want preventive lifestyle counseling. That's wonderful. Of the other 90 percent, about half are people who come with routine conditions: hayfever, arthritis, chronic sinus conditions, and digestive problems. In those instances, what I provide is truly alternative medicine. I tell people to do things *in place* of what regular doctors would tell them. In these cases, the conventional treatments are last resorts, in my opinion. They're what you do after simple methods have failed. Unfortunately, medical students don't learn the simple methods.

The other half of that group are people with overwhelming diseases. I see a lot of people with cancer. I see a lot of people with very serious medical conditions for which there are no easy answers and often no answers at all in conventional medicine. In those instances, a lot of what I do is complementary medicine. These people end up doing some combinations of regular treatment and alternative treatment. Often the two work very well together. Virtually all patients who come to see me have been through conventional medicine and have not been helped. Many of them have been hurt by their encounters with regular doctors. They've been hurt financially, or physically, or emotionally, or all of the above.

They tend to be people who are intelligent, educated, and highly motivated to take responsibility for their own well-being, and I like working with them. They are a self-selected group. They're looking for information. When they get it, they're going to run with it and apply it. They just want to know what to do.

I am alarmed at the numbers of patients who come to see me who have been hexed by doctors. I use that term very advisedly. There is a formal term, "medical hexing," used mostly by anthropologists and psychotherapists who have studied voodoo practices and shamanistic practices in cultures where malevolent witch doctors curse people, often at the behest of an enemy. The person goes home and stops eating, stops interacting with relatives and family, lies in bed, weakens, and in some cases, dies. There have been many documented cases of that sort of thing. It's called voodoo death.

I think an exact analog of that process goes on every day in doctors' offices and hospitals in this country, and I see the results of it. Occasionally, doctors hex patients in anger because they dislike them, but that's very rare. For example, I had a woman patient in her mid-fifties who had metastatic ovarian cancer and who was in a very bad relationship with her oncologist. She kept telling the oncologist that she was going to beat the odds of this disease, and he kept telling her she wasn't. Finally one day she said, "Look, I am going to beat this thing," and he said, "The only way you're not going to die of your cancer is if you get hit by a truck." At that point she got angry enough to fire him and find another oncologist, which she should have done long before.

That's rare. Much more commonly I see situations in which doctors have completely unthinkingly and unconsciously said things to patients that convey the message that healing is not possible. Probably the doctors wouldn't even remember saying them. They're offhand, haphazard remarks, yet for the patients, even years later, they burn in their minds and obstruct the activation of internal healing processes.

A patient came to me from Vancouver, a fifty-three-year-old man with a three-year history of urinary problems that he had ignored. His wife came in to see me, and he stayed out in the driveway in his car. She said he was so terrified of doctors that he couldn't bring himself to see another one. I listened to her first, and then I went out and persuaded him to come in. He had finally gone to a urologist at the University of British Columbia, and it had turned out he had prostate cancer already metastatic to bones of the pelvis. That's a poor prognosis. Surgery, chemotherapy, and radiation were not options. The only treatment they offered was hormones to slow the growth of the cancer.

He was sent away with that. My immediate sense of this man was that he was in total terror. He had seized on visualization as the thing that was going to save him and was spending two hours a day intensely visualizing his immune cells dealing with the cancer. But in the meantime, he was a chain smoker. I asked him about the smoking and out came this story. He said that six months earlier, he had been at the University of British Columbia when the urologist had given him the diagnosis. He had asked, "Should I stop smoking?" The doctor said to him, "At this point, why bother?"

Now I think if the doctor even remembered saying that, he would say he was doing the patient a favor—trying to spare him further trouble. But what the patient heard was, "You are going to die soon." I think that's exactly equivalent to a hex placed by a shaman. Here is a priest of technological medicine sitting in his temple uttering a pronouncement of doom. That was the source of the patient's terror, and the reason why he could not do anything constructive to change his lifestyle. In fact, there is no way to know if that patient is going to die soon. You can find many examples of metastatic prostate cancer in which patients either explicably or inexplicably have lived for long periods of time in relatively good health. For one reason or another, their immune systems managed to check the cancer.

Why do doctors do this sort of thing? My sense is that it reveals a deep pessimism on the part of doctors about healing. Many of them don't believe that people get better. Why don't they believe it? Examples of people getting better are all over the place. As a result of the work that I do, I get case reports from all over the world of cures of supposedly incurable conditions. In many cases, I've had a chance to meet the patients and verify the stories to my satisfaction. What these reports testify to is the human capacity to get better, to heal, which should be obvious. You can see it in yourself, you can see it in your dog, you can see it in your plants, you can see it in everything. Nature tends to heal itself when it's disturbed. Why don't doctors see that?

There are two reasons, I think. One is that their training doesn't show it to them. The whole medical curriculum is about disease. There's nothing about health, nothing about healing. Why isn't there a course in remission to balance the course in pathology? There's nothing. Furthermore, when doctors get into hospitals, their actual experience of sick people is with a very skewed sample. They see the very sick, many of whom do not recover.

Such limited experience breeds an incredible lack of belief in the human body's ability to repair itself. Clearly, we have a self-repair system, a healing system, something we share with all of nature. We share it with rivers, with plants. Everything has this capacity to heal itself when disturbed. It's a universal tendency to seek equilibrium.

Years ago, when I was an undergraduate, I worked on the Harvard newspaper, and I interviewed a proto-ecologist who was studying rivers. I remember his telling me—it made a great impression—that rivers were living organisms. It was a novel concept to me. He said that rivers had a variety of systems to handle a certain amount of pollution. These included the bacteria and plants that lived in the river, and the oxygenation of water running through turbulent areas. He said that if you didn't put too much stuff into a river, it could detoxify itself and get rid of it. But if you overloaded it, you gradually poisoned those systems, and then the river died. However, if you stopped putting toxins in, eventually levels would drop to a point where those natural healing systems would revive.

I believe all aspects of nature share that capacity. I was taught in medical school that atherosclerosis, the deposition of cholesterol in arteries, especially in coronary arteries, is an irreversible process. Why should it be irreversible? Why, if you stop the cause of arterial pollution, can't the body find mechanisms to clean it up? Now there is evidence that it can do precisely that.

Medical doctors are continuously taught that things can't get better, that things can't heal, and they give this belief back to patients. In my experience, shamans who serve as healers do much better. Regardless of what methods they use—from sucking out invisible darts to giving people hallucinogenic plants—they are master psychotherapists. Shamans are especially good at taking the belief that people project onto them and reflecting it back in the service of healing. That's what doctors should be doing. All this belief is being projected onto them, but too often what doctors send back is a negative message. "You can't get better. You'll have to live with it. There's nothing we can do for you. You'll have to have surgery. You'll have to take this drug for the rest of your life."

This has to change. If we could get change in medicine—because it is so central in our society—I believe we would see positive change in many other areas of our culture.

The medical profession has painted itself into a corner by preferring treatments that are so dangerous, so expensive, and so reliant on technology. It has also separated itself from nature. Doctors fail to see that healing is fundamentally a natural process. They are unable to use the power that people give them in the service of healing. We can change this situation. The greening of the pharmacopoeia is an important first step. The new medicine that is coming into being can help heal our society and the entire planet.

The Role of Herbs
in Integrative Medicine

Tieraona Low Dog

Dr. Tieraona (Ta-row-nay) Low Dog is a dazzling expression of the transformation under way in health care. Among the most dynamic and eloquent advocates of plant medicine, she serves as a member of the White House Commission on Complementary and Alternative Medicine Policy. As one of the country's leading experts on botanical medicine and integrative approaches to health, she chairs the influential U.S. Pharmacopoeia Dietary Supplements—Botanicals Expert Committee, which evaluates the clinical evidence of commonly used herbs. She can rap biochemistry with the best of them.

But what makes her even more impressive is that she began her work as the Herb Lady of Las Cruces, New Mexico, with a three-week waiting list. "I didn't go to medical school to become a doctor," she says. "I saw myself as a doctor who did not have enough diagnostic capabilities or the knowledge/ability to have really powerful medicine when people needed it."

She grew up on the Lakota Sioux reservation in South Dakota, where her father's mother was a midwife and his father a healer. She studied with a Paiute family that tended sheep in the Arizona desert, and she also learned from her Irish-American grandmother in Kansas, a Jamaican midwife, and her Korean martial arts instructor (she has a third-degree black belt and has won national tae kwon do championships). She apprenticed as a midwife for more than five years and served as president of the American Herbalist Guild.

The Herb Lady's turning point occurred in Las Cruces when a Mexican man came to her with a very sick baby. She gave him herbs and money for Tylenol but told him he really needed to see a doctor. Four days later he returned to thank her before going back to Mexico with his dead baby. "I felt like the world just stopped at that moment," she recalls. "What if I could have done more? I'll always feel responsible for that baby's death." That's when she decided to go to medical school.

Go she did, despite having only an eighth-grade formal education and a general equivalency diploma, as well as being a single mom who was home-schooling her son. Today she serves as medical director for the Tree House Center of Integrative Medicine in Albuquerque, New Mexico, a family medicine practice treating women and children. She is assistant clinical professor in the Department of Family and Community Medicine at the University of New Mexico School of Medicine and clinical lecturer for the Department of Medicine at the University of Arizona School of Medicine in Tucson. With her herbalist husband, she is designing continuing medical education learning modules on botanical medicine.

Tieraona was named by Time magazine as an Innovator in Alternative Medicine for 2001 and is a past recipient of the Martina de la Cruz Medal for her human rights work with indigenous people and remedies.

❀   ❀   ❀

IT'S STAGGERING WHEN YOU LOOK at the millions of children on Ritalin. It's staggering when you look at the millions of people who are on antidepressants, the millions of people who get bypass surgery as they eat their hamburgers all the way to the surgeon's office. It is staggering when one thinks that the tobacco companies are now advertising their good deeds as part of their settlement and at the same time targeting Hispanic teenage women because their studies have shown that they're the group that smokes the least.

So now we have José and Josephina Camel in New Mexico selling cancer. It is staggering when you think of tuberculosis in Russia, but you don't have to go that far. You just have to go to the inner city or to the Indian reservations of the United States to find it. Obesity used to be a disease of old age. Old people got type II diabetes. Now we see it in children twelve or thirteen years of age, especially among many Native American youth. Is this health care? Are we doing a good job? I don't think so.

And is the answer simply herbs? I would argue it is not. If we simply re-place a drug with an herb, we have missed the opportunity for true healing to take place. There's a lot that we can do with herbs, but if you reduce these plants to merely their constituents, synthesize them, reproduce them, and use them as drugs, you have not changed anything. Dietary supplements and botanicals constitute an industry worth more than $14 billion a year, but in-stead of really getting to the root of our health problems and promoting well-ness, we're looking for things inside of a pill. Plants are seeds and they grow. They teach us about the cycles of life and death.

If you took some of those children on Ritalin and put them in a garden planting seeds, tending the soil, and working on their own inner landscapes, you might find that they would be fine without their medication. My own son was diagnosed with attention-deficit/hyperactivity disorder and went the route of Ritalin. We later home-schooled him, brought him into martial arts, did all the things we thought were good to nurture his soul. When he was eighteen he said to me, "Mom, I appreciate everything you did for me, but the thing I appreciate the most is that you finally recognized there was nothing ever wrong with me."

Pharmaceutical companies drive research in this country. Herbs are nat-ural substances. They cannot be patented. There is no incentive for research. Nobody's going to pay for it. If you're a large company, why are you going to spend $50 million to study echinacea when anybody can sell it at the health food store? Heck, you can grow it in your yard.

There is a misperception that herbs have no value because they have not been researched. Some have been researched, just not in this country, and we will probably never do extensive research on herbs because of what drives medicine.

When is enough evidence enough? I hear this litany all the time: You need more evidence. But when we bring the evidence, it's still not enough. Saw palmetto is a good example. If you're a man and you live long enough you'll probably get an enlarged prostate. Let's say you come to see me as a patient, and you're a sixty-five-year-old gentleman with a limited income and your Medicare is through an HMO and you have very mild symptoms of enlarged prostate. Your blood pressure is normal. What's on formulary is a blood pressure—lowering medication that will also shrink the prostate, making it easier to urinate more freely. You must take it at night so you don't get dizzy and fall down because your blood pressure's through the floor. You take it at night to prevent orthostatic hypotension. But your blood pressure is normal. Why can't I prescribe saw palmetto? Saw palmetto works. We've had a meta-analysis in the *Journal of the American Medical Association* (*JAMA*), the bible of Western medical research, that says it works.

The United States Pharmacopoeia—I chair the Dietary Supplements—Botanicals Expert Committee—gave a positive monograph. Even the urologists said, "Gee, this stuff looks pretty good." A man can get his medication for a $2 copayment at the pharmacy, but if he wants saw palmetto, it's $28 down at the health food store. At what point is there enough research? Twenty-eight trials? Meta-analysis in *JAMA*? The United States Pharmacopoeia saying it works? And yet it's still not covered because we see it as CAM (complementary and alternative medicine) and there is no pharmaceutical company lobbying for it to be covered. There's no pharmaceutical company handing out notepads and pens touting saw palmetto to the residents in medical school. That's an inequity.

Saw palmetto offers men a safe, appropriate, and effective treatment for a very common problem. When you're a sixty-five- or seventy-five-year-old gentleman, I don't want to give you something that lowers your blood pressure and increases your risk of falls, because what if you fall when you're seventy-five years of age and you break your hip? Then we have even more trouble. For mild symptoms of enlarged prostate, why isn't saw palmetto covered?

What about glucosamine? It's been used for more than twenty years in Europe and helps arthritis. Arthritis, though not life threatening, sure costs a lot of money to treat. Now we've got glucosamine that has been systematically reviewed, with sixteen trials showing that it works, and four trials showing that it works as well as the best nonsteroidal we have to offer. It doesn't cause ulcers or renal failure. A three-year study published in the *Lancet* showed that glucosamine may reverse osteoarthritis. We don't prescribe it. It's not paid for. It's not covered. Why?

One has to question at what point something becomes a medicine. At what point do we offer the best treatments that are safe, effective, and available? Why should people who are economically disadvantaged not be entitled to use products that are often safer and just as efficacious because they're not covered by HMOs, Medicare, or Medicaid? We can't even get food stamps to cover multivitamins.

I like garlic. Garlic has been primarily studied for its benefits in lowering cholesterol, but its use for more than twenty-five centuries was actually as an antimicrobial. They used to call it Russian penicillin because it was so valued in poorer countries for its antimicrobial activity. Albert Schweitzer said there was never a case of dysentery that he could not effectively treat with garlic. Louis Pasteur was the first one to document its antiseptic properties. Japanese researchers have found that garlic, even when heated to temperatures that exceed 100 degrees centigrade, remains antimicrobial against the notorious E-coli 0157. Garlic may also be effective against salmonella, vibrio cholera, and giardia, major gut pathogens that cause terrible and often life-threatening diarrhea.

Garlic also benefits heart health. These days it seems that everybody is going out and getting a heart bypass. My grandmother is in her nineties and it was recommended that she have bypass surgery. She said no thank you. Surgeons would saw open her chest and when it's all done, stitch her back up like a turkey. She's in her nineties! She would never recover from that type of surgery. Trust her to know. Trust her to know that she's old and that's not the way she wants to live her life. I did say to my grandma, "Hey, grandma, how about you get a book by Dean Ornish. It's a great book. It talks about eating food a little differently, maybe, than the way you have thought about." I get a little angry because her doctor has never talked to her about this. She gets $411 a month from Social Security, from which she has to pay for everything. She has Medicare and her cholesterol-lowering medication costs more than $120 a month. Nobody has ever, ever said one word to her about her diet. She went and got that Dean Ornish book and this little old lady in Kansas got so excited. "What is T-O-F-U? Can I get that in Kansas?"

Nutrition is so important, and it's a part of Western medicine to which we pay little attention. "Let thy food be thy medicine and thy medicine be thy food." Much of the food we eat today makes us sick. What do we expect? We're going to have generations of people lined up for bypass surgery when Burger King is in the high school and the elementary schools sell soda pop so they can earn money for the band.

I do find it amusing that people buy ground-up broccoli in a capsule and pay $ 30 a bottle for it when they could have just gotten a bunch of it and eaten it for dinner.

Let's get back to garlic. Physicians argue it only reduces cholesterol by about 10 percent. What else does it do besides reduce your cholesterol? It makes platelets less likely to aggregate. We want your platelets to be a little less sticky so you don't get a clot going somewhere that will harm or kill you. Garlic lowers cholesterol, makes your blood pressure go down a little, about 5 to 7 percent, and a four-year study in Germany showed that it actually reverses atherosclerotic plaque in arteries. Garlic! Garlic is food. It's medicine. It's cheap. Eat it!

The leading cause of blindness in the United States is from diabetes, diabetic retinopathy. Bilberries, European blueberries, have a protective effect on the capillaries of the eyes. This is important for me to know working in a community with many Hispanic and Native American individuals, many of whom have diabetes. Blueberries might help protect their eyes and kidneys.

Should bilberries only be taken ground up, concentrated, and standardized in a pill? Not necessarily. It is very healthy to eat them fresh. A standardized reductionist drug model of herbs and foods takes us away, again, from healthy living: eating organic fruits and vegetables. Seventy percent of your diet should be based on plants: whole grains, fruits, and vegetables. Plants have a role to play in promoting wellness, and I believe that they can be used in many ways to treat many conditions.

Echinacea is another herb I'm a fan of. It was one of the most popular anti-infectives in the United States until 1920. We know that its prime effect is enhancing the body's ability to fight off upper-respiratory infections. One thing we seem to have forgotten today is that we didn't survive a million years on this planet by never getting sick. Our bodies are strong. We're strong. Letting your body get sick every once in a while is a good thing. Learning from illness can be a powerful way to grow.

Sometimes it's okay to do nothing, to quit doing stuff. Quit automatically giving women hormones when they go through menopause, as though we are all diseased. My God, just let us be. I find it interesting that well-informed and educated women go in and ask some twenty-five-year-old male doctor, "What should I do?" What the hell would he know about what you should do? You can take hormones or you can not take hormones. You decide, but just know that menopause is like everything else in our life: It's a time of opportunity. It's a transition. It's a change. Illness is transformative. I am grateful for antibiotics. I'm grateful for emergency surgery. I'm grateful for all of the gifts that Western medicine has brought, but it is not the only game in town, and may not be the best game in town for some of the problems that we're trying to deal with today.

I'm hoping for a greening of medicine, and I think plants are symbolic of that. They're a piece of it, but if we just look to herbs as a replacement for drugs without doing anything else, we've missed this opportunity to really change our lives for the better. "Paradise" comes from the Persian word for garden. The plants themselves are transformative.

Joseph Campbell said that it is in the garden that wonders are revealed. And I'd say that that's true. A garden is one place where you can hear your inner voice, in the quiet. We all have the power within us, just like the seed, to make change.

Community Herbalism
in Modern Health Care

Christopher Hobbs

Christopher Hobbs is an internationally renowned figure in the field of botanical medicine. As a fourth-generation botanist, he comes from a lineage of green genes. He has thirty-four years' experience as a clinical herbalist and also practices as a licensed acupuncturist. He has written, cowritten, or edited twenty-four books on health and herbal medicine, including Herbal Remedies for Dummies, Natural Liver Therapy, Botanical Safety Handbook, *and the* Peterson Field Guide to Western Medicinal Plants and Herbs.

Chris has a uniquely compelling vision of how to integrate the dynamic resurgence of herbalism into the contemporary medical and social landscape. He has an astute and precise understanding of when the use of herbs is appropriate and when it is not. His repertoire draws from a diversity of rich traditions, and he is firmly grounded in modern science and biochemistry.

But the exceptional quality of Chris's mastery of plant medicine arises from his intimate connection with the earth. More than that, his love of plants and the land have compelled him to ruminate on what it means to develop an ethic that places plants, people, and health on an equal footing. He is rebirthing lapsed traditions of bioregional herbal wisdom that give people a sense of place. His vision is encouraging individuals and local communities to take control of their own health care and renew their bonds to the natural world in ways that will assure both the public health and the vitality of the ecosystems on which it depends.

*   *   *

I'VE BEEN A PRACTICING HERBALIST for thirty-three years, and my maternal grandmother and great-grandmother were also herbalists. My father was a professor of botany, and his father was a professor of botany. So I didn't have much choice in the matter; I had to study herbs. I'm also a licensed acupuncturist, and I've had a clinical practice for many years. Recently I moved to Davis, California, in order to go back to school to get a Ph.D. in pharmacology and toxicology. My reason for doing that is that I want to help people get off drugs and help get more natural medicines into hospital formularies, and I think working inside the system might be a good way to help accomplish that.

I'm very interested in developing the concept of bioregional herbalism— interacting and developing a relationship with healing plants that grow in one's own area. Of course that includes native plants, but also many plants that may have originated in some other place and have made themselves quite at home in new locales. Sometimes ornamentals planted for their beauty in one place turn out to be valued for their medicinal properties in other cultures. For example, the small purple fruits of a common street tree all over central California called Waxed Tree Privet (*Ligustrum lucidum*) are one of the major kidney tonics used in Chinese medicine. In fact, one could walk outside anywhere in California and look at the weeds, trees, and ornamentals, and it would turn out that most of them are used for medicine somewhere in some culture of the world. So, using one's local plants can actually involve broadening one's medicinal horizons.

The sales of pharmaceutical drugs in this country currently generate $160 billion per year. The sinus decongestant Claritin and two similar drugs alone bring in more in sales in this country than the entire herbal industry. The top-selling drug categories are antidepressants (about $12.5 billion in sales, at about $73 for the average prescription), ulcer medications, cholesterol-lowering drugs, antibiotics, anti-arthritics, anti-hypertensives, and oral diabetes drugs.

It's been the most profitable sector of the economy every year since 1982. Drug company profits averaged about three times the norm for Fortune 500 companies. Surprisingly few innovative new drugs are developed by companies' research and development, and drug companies don't often focus on drugs that could really save millions of lives, such as anti-malarials, because there's no money in drugs for the poor. The pharmaceutical companies also get generous tax credits and spend enormously on ad campaigns, as we all know, since their ads are everywhere.

These days one hears a great deal about the need for "evidence-based medicine," the importance of human studies showing the clinical effectiveness and safety of the medicines that we take. Herbs are often criticized because there supposedly aren't any studies showing their effectiveness and safety. But when you analyze reliable data you find that maybe only 25 percent of pharmaceutical drugs have good, solid clinical evidence proving their effectiveness, and only a much smaller percentage have had their long-term safety rigorously tested. Many drugs are prescribed off label, that is, approved for a certain use but prescribed for something else, further increasing safety risks and uncertainty about effectiveness. Ninety million Americans take drugs daily, about one in three, and drug side effects account for probably over one hundred thousand deaths per year just in U.S. hospitals.

Perhaps sixty-five million people in this country use herbs for health. Maybe about a quarter of those use pharmaceutical drugs and herbs together. How do drugs and herbs interact? There's a lot that we don't know, but there are very, very few actual reports of negative herb-drug interactions. There's a lot of theoretical speculation, but very few actual reports of herbs interfering with drugs. This is not a major safety issue.

Why can't we get more herbs and herb products on hospital formularies? Many herbs such as St. John's wort, ginkgo, ginseng, saw palmetto, garlic, and echinacea have good clinical research showing their effectiveness and safety. They usually have about half the side effects of the comparable pharmaceutical drug that is used for similar conditions, at one quarter of the cost. So why aren't we prescribing these for the first line of treatment in milder cases? The United States spends more on health care than any other nation in the world, even with forty-three million people who don't have health insurance. Using more herbal medicine makes sense medically and financially.

Many herbalists are wary of standardization: using solvents to purify a certain fraction of the plant and turning it into more of a drug than an herb, rather than using the whole herb as a tea. But we need some form of standardization, because consumers need to be sure of a product's quality and identity. The herb industry has been criticized for being largely unregulated. The FDA has a lot to do. It has to regulate medical devices and pharmaceutical drugs, and a lot of other things. We need some form of self-regulation in the herb industry, and we do have some, and it is getting better.

Standardization simply implies having a consistent product so you know that when you purchase an herb, it's the right herb and it's going to have a certain level of quality and consistency. The traditional village or community herbalist who knows patients personally and who has been trained in how to use herbs, when to harvest an herb at its peak for optimum potency, what part to harvest, where to go to harvest it, how to process it, how to extract it, how to dry it, and so on, does in fact assure a form of standardization.

Also, in traditional systems such as Chinese medicine or Ayurveda, the individual patient is looked at in the context of the family, the whole society, and the larger environment of the natural world. These systems look at how internal organs change with changing seasons, how we're more susceptible to dryness diseases in the fall and to wetness or dampness diseases in the spring, for example. They use methods of pulse and tongue diagnosis and try to tailor the herbs or the herb formula to the specific patient in a specific context. This is a form of sophisticated "standardization," but at the level of community herbalism. This is an herbalism that may vary community by community; it's bioregional herbalism.

But if one goes to Thrifty's or Long's and buys a ginkgo extract, the leaves were probably growth in North Carolina. They were most likely then shipped to China to be extracted, and then shipped to Germany to be tested, because the Germans have the best high-performance liquid chromatography technology with which to check the purity of compounds. Then the product was manufactured and shipped to this country. This is a much wider web and though it involves more modern technology, the quality of the original material is actually harder to determine. If you buy a Chinese patent medicine, it might have been manufactured a few years ago, the pills are often coated with dye and sugar, and they sometimes contain heavy metals, including perhaps unacceptable levels of mercury and lead.

We need some form of standardization and regulation, but if you're using the plants directly from your region, and you are working with a well-trained traditional herbalist, then you don't have all of these problems. Better yet, learn how to use herbs yourself and discover the healing properties of the plants that are growing in your yard and the fields and forests around you.

High-tech uniform standardization simply can't take into account that different plants vary in strength depending on where they're growing and what time of the year the plant is harvested. Experienced herbalists know most roots are best harvested in the fall, barks in the spring and fall, when the sap is moving in the bark, flowers just before buds open, and seeds when they're green but not dried in the sun, for example. That's real herbal knowledge.

Some might argue that type of herbalism is a thing of the past, but it's alive and well. There's a community called Village Homes in Davis, California, an intentional community based on permaculture principles that was built in the early 1970s. When you walk through that community, you see medicinal plants planted along the pathways, all kinds of edible and medicinal plants incorporated right into the design of the community. We designed and built two community gardens in Santa Cruz over the last ten years that we called "the living farmacy" based on the principles of bioregional herbalism. Our centers had a lot of students coming and going, and my students are carrying on the tradition there. We do apprenticeships and classes and train people how to use medicinal plants in both Santa Cruz and Davis. We also developed a similar community garden in Williams, Oregon. Many other herbal centers are actively training herbalists throughout North America.

In Santa Cruz we have a very large and active community of people who are studying medicinal plants, and it includes an acupuncture school for those who want to study traditional Chinese medicine. But the garden has been the center, and we also have an extraction plant developed by my students to produce the medicines that are used in locals clinics. Why can't we have a medicinal plant garden in the center of each community? Each community could have a school that trains people how to take care of their own health using these simple plant medicines, which are so safe and effective and have been used for thousands of years.

Get to know your habitat, your climate, and what medicinal plants can grow there. In Williams, California, for example, there are winter freezes, a nice riparian zone, and a hardwood canopy that is deal for ginseng, goldenseal, black cohosh, blue cohosh. So we planted those famous eastern medicinal plants, which can now be used along with a lot of native plants from Williams's own bioregional area in the local herbal pharmacopoeia. Many of the most popular herbal medicines such as ginseng, goldenseal, St. John's wort, and echinacea can be easily grown in your own garden. This is direct medicine. If you're growing echinacea, for example, and you feel a cold coming on, simply go out in your garden and pick half a leaf, chew it up, and swallow it. This is commonly done in many cultures.

Tremendous healing energy is produced in interaction with plants through smelling, tasting, and ingesting small amounts. The best healing comes through our relationship with the plants themselves.

It's not hard to learn how to grow plants and to harvest herbs by shade-drying them carefully, as quickly as possible with a warm current of air, and then putting them in airtight jars to make tea later. Nor is it hard to make an effective medicinal tea by taking one part dried plant to ten parts water and either infusing or decocting it, or to learn to make your own herbal tinctures. Incorporate useful plants in your garden and around your house, or even in a planter box. You can grow almost any medicinal plant. These medicines can be highly effective.

If we can each learn twenty local plants—cultivated and wild plants and weeds in our area—we can cover most conditions, most symptoms, most ailments that we might come across in our daily lives. Find twenty local plants, make a connection with them, learn more about them, and start to use them. Be your own bioregional herbalist.

Relationships Are the Best Medicine

Jeanne Achterberg

For over three decades, Dr. Jeanne Achterberg has been awakening the health care field to the fundamental interconnections among mind, body, and spirit. She has shown an exceptional capacity to dissolve the illusory boundaries that have kept these dimensions separate in medicine.

She is adept at the clear, precise, linear discipline that science so often requires. Yet at the same time she skillfully integrates the mysteries of mind and spirit, incorporating intuitive knowing, creativity, and the wisdom of the heart into the redefinition of medicine and healing.

She began her work with the renowned oncologist O. Carl Simonton and his wife, who were helping cancer patients fight malignancies by drawing on visualization, attitudinal healing, and the support of other patients. The author of the classic book Imagery in Healing: Shamanism and Modern Medicine, *she is perhaps best known for her pioneering work using guided imagery to effect healing. When she began this kind of work in the 1960s, it bordered on medical heresy. Today it is standard practice in hospitals all over the world.*

Twelve years ago Jeanne wrote the landmark book Woman as Healer, *tracing the role of women in health care from prehistory to the present. The conceptual framework she provided proved to be prescient. When she wrote the book in 1980, over 80 percent of health care workers in the United States were women, yet most had limited opportunity and authority. Between 1970 and 1999, women's enrollment in medical schools increased from 6 percent to 42 percent. The American Medical Association predicts that by 2010, nearly one-third of all physicians will be women.*

Jeanne has been a mind-body therapy trainer for health care professionals throughout the world and has also served populations in crisis, including refugees in

Kosovo and Macedonia. She has won countless awards in recognition of her immense contributions to medicine. Time *magazine featured her in 2001 as one of the six leading innovators in alternative medicine of our era.*

Most recently, Jeanne personally confronted the life-and-death challenge of can-cer. Diagnosed with a rare melanoma of the eye, she chronicled the story of her own recovery using alternative therapies in the book Lightning at the Gate. *In this fiercely courageous memoir, she tells how receiving the prayers of her community helped heal her, a kind of collective, nonlocal approach she calls transpersonal medicine.*

❧   ❧   ❧

WE ARE IN CRISIS. In medicine we are in an economic crisis, but one that goes far beyond the problem of not being able to pay for medical care. We are in an environmental crisis, but it goes beyond the abuse and the neglect of our environment. Fundamentally, these are side effects of a greater crisis, and that is our failure to respect men, women, and children, a failure to honor human-ity, to honor life, and a failure to ask with each thought, "Is this life-giving? Is this life sustaining? Or is this destructive?"

What is the evidence that honoring human values makes any difference in the health of a planet, the health of a community? Truth comes before us in many guises—as poetry, art, music, and science. We can draw from scientists, ancient wisdom traditions, artists, poets, or mystics; they can all provide us in their own ways with rich imagery of the human connection, the centrality of human relationship and of a universe in which we are all connected by an ineffable, invisible matrix.

It's a trellis upon which humanity weaves itself into an immense and dy-namic tapestry. Each life, each soul, the essence of each being is a point of light in the cloth. Like the web of a tireless spider, the warps and strands gracefully dance and shape and reshape in multidimensional space. It folds upon itself like a night-blooming flower in the path of a full moon. Think of this cloth as

the consciousness of humankind, grafting itself upon the source of its own divine origin, countless filaments connecting.

In some traditions it is said that when two lights, two souls, the essence
of two human beings bond, energy is released, great quantities of light and
sound are released, and the nature of each is changed forever. We merge with
each other and with the source from which we came. According to these teachings, when we profoundly connect with another human being, we not only
polish our souls in theirs, we may even release light and energy. And what
do we know from poetry, from listening and from paying attention? We know
that perhaps medicine is simply a life raft and we human beings hold onto one
another in a great sea. James Baldwin said, "The moment we cease to hold each
other, the moment we lose faith in one another, the sea engulfs us, the light
goes out."

What can we say about human relationship on a level that's concrete and
scientific? Well, we can say that relationships are very effective stress buffers.
Study after study shows that people in relationships have increased immune
function, decreased wound healing time, lower sympathetic nervous system
activity. We know that it's hard to kill a married man, even if he's not really
wild about his wife. We know that women who have girlfriends live forever.
So science marches on. According to research, relationships are a panacea that
decreases the incidence of death from all major causes. Imagine the value of
the stock of a pharmaceutical firm that could make that claim about one of its
products. Apparently being together on this life raft in this sea is a panacea.
So relationships might be the best medicine. People in a relationship who can
identify a supportive community are at less risk for complications from virtually everything you can name: tuberculosis, psychiatric disorders, arthritis,
high blood pressure, and so on.

I had a rather interesting, challenging event several years ago that brought
me to my knees in terms of what I thought I knew about medicine and what
I thought I knew about relationship. I was working in the refugee camps in
Macedonia right after the Kosovo war and was there for quite a while in the
biggest camp. Sometimes there were as many as 20,000 people coming and
going in that camp. One day, during the biggest migration, I stood in the

middle of thousands and thousands of these gentle people. When I made eye contact with thousands of them, I felt for the first time in my life what it was like to be part of the whole human family. Suffering connects our hearts.

On the way home after that epiphany I prayed and prayed that I would develop a new vision. I felt in the very marrow of my bones that the insular way in which I was living my life and looking at the world no longer served. Then, within weeks of getting home, I went blind. Be careful what you pray for. I was diagnosed with a very large and rapidly growing ocular melanoma, and my life expectancy was probably in the months, given the size of the melanoma and my general condition. The irony of all of this is that I'd been in the alternative medicine field for a long time, and I'd been a faculty member at Southwestern Medical School for a long time as well, so I knew both realms of medicine intimately. Neither of them could offer a cure. The alternative medicine people wouldn't even see me, they said, until I had my eye removed, and that was something that I could not bring myself to do. It's not cured, incidentally, but as Mark Twain once said, the reports of my death have been greatly exaggerated.

Thanks to Larry and Barbara Dossey and many other friends, prayer circles began to be formed for me all over the world, and they continue to function. I must have the most prayed-for eye on the face of the earth. After all that, as a scientist, I felt absolutely compelled to begin to study healing bonds. I started thinking about what the bonds might actually be. The first type of bond I call transpersonal. It's what I could palpably feel when people far away were praying for me, for example. This is what we now call distant intentionality. Transpersonal bonds are invisible energy-based links that tie us to the healing web of all life and consciousness.

The second level of healing bond is one that was very difficult for me to discuss until I had the experience in Kosovo. It's what I would call a soul connection. Anyone who's ever been with a loved one in crisis probably knows what a soul connection is. It takes us beyond ego to a sense of unity and connection with someone else.

The third level of healing is touch, flesh-to-flesh connection, as found in massage, the power of holding, and therapeutic touch. There is an abundance of research showing that touch heals. I've listened to a lot of very old and very sick people who tell me they really still need to be touched, and many still want to make love. Perhaps it is in times when we are in greatest crisis—be it physical, mental, or spiritual—that we need to touch each other most. Any of us who have ever nursed a baby know that far more than milk is being transmitted in that act.

The next level of healing bond is the community web. There is so much research, some of it going back thirty and forty years, showing that the community web of family, friends, work, and other support networks is profoundly healing. I love the research about a community in Pennsylvania, the Rosetta community, that was full of Italians who had the nerve to smoke, drink, sit around, not exercise, get fat, and astonish the epidemiologists because they had only half the cardiac disease of all the neighboring communities. The prediction was made that once they migrated away from their family roots, they would lose their cardiovascular advantage, and sure enough they did.

Now the healing bond that is perhaps most intriguing is the bond of love. Is it lifesaving? Many of the survivors of the most dire and difficult circumstances say it is. Victor Frankl, for example, said that when he was in the concentration camps, he clung to his wife's image and would not have endured if he'd known she was dead.

So what do people in a health crisis want? What is it we can do as health care providers, as intelligent consumers? Epidemiological research from all over the world shows that people basically go into the health care system to get relief from suffering and to get information, but every single piece of evidence points to the fact that when they are also given sympathy, compassion, and understanding, all of the medicines that are prescribed tend to work better. Is this so difficult for us to understand?

I would like to share with you some remarks from someone much wiser than I am about the nature of compassion, human relationships, and love. The great mystic, scientist, and Jesuit Teilhard de Chardin said, "Love is the free and imaginative outpouring of the spirit over all unexplored paths. It links those who love in bonds that unite but do not confound, causing them to discover in their mutual contact an exaltation capable of arousing in the heart of their being all that they possess in uniqueness and power. . . . Someday, after we have mastered the winds, the waves, the tides and gravity, we shall harness for good the energies of love, and then, for the second time in the history of the world, we will have discovered fire."

Mothering on the Front Lines: Protecting Kids

Peggy O'Mara

Peggy O'Mara is the mother of all mothers. As the editor and publisher of Mothering *magazine for the past twenty-three years, she has not only chronicled the renaissance of natural parenting and childbirth, she has lived it.*

Peggy herself is the mother of four young adults, now aged nineteen to twenty-eight, and her own experiences led to her emergence as a trusted source of information and dialogue. She has been the fulcrum for millions of women who are reevaluating conventional medicine's medicalization of child bearing and rearing and rediscovering the ancient healing wisdom of women.

The author of Natural Family Living *and* Having a Baby Naturally, *she also acts as editor of* Vaccinations: The Issue of Our Times. *Her early work questioning the safety and necessity of vaccinations prefigured current debates about the possible association of rising autism rates with mercury-based vaccines. It has also deepened questions about such questionable bioterrorism responses as mass smallpox vaccinations among U.S. health care workers, whose general refusal to participate in the program has highlighted the kinds of credible concerns Peggy has been raising for decades. Peggy also embodies the movement to resist the commodification of childhood, both in her personal life and in her articulate and passionate advocacy.*

❀   ❀   ❀

MANY OF US ARE CONCERNED with living in a less toxic environment. We eat organic food and try to maintain a nontoxic home, yet we may
be hitting our kids, or allowing them to be injected with poisons in certain
vaccines, or letting their minds be colonized by commercialism. These are actually things that we can do something about, that we can really have an impact on.

The tendency in our culture, starting at birth, is to overpower our own
natures. Pregnant women are not encouraged to trust their own natures. Pregnancy is seen as a disease. We don't appreciate birth as normal, so there is, from
the very beginning, an attempt to dominate our very natures. I believe that
when we do this, we do violence to ourselves and to nature in general. These
are the first intrusions of power, technology, materialism, and commercialism
into our inherent natures. Throughout our lives society makes us feel as if we're
not good enough as we are, so I think we need to translate our environmental
and social consciousness into daily life. Let's clean up the toxins and disarm
the world by beginning with ourselves, the only person we really have any
control over.

The ritual of birth is supposed to be a template for the future, so that we
imprint upon our culture and later follow its traditions. But what babies often
imprint to in our culture is drugs. About 80 percent of women take drugs
during childbirth and about 30 percent give birth surgically. Often a baby's
first experience is to have his or her body flooded by drugs. Research in Sweden shows that babies who have been exposed to barbiturates during labor
have more of a tendency to be addicted to barbiturates in adulthood. We never
hear about this. In our society we value freedom of choice. Women want to
be able to choose to take drugs or not in childbirth. But what is the effect on
the baby of the drugs in the mother? When drugs are administered to children, the dosage is based on their weight, but the dose of drugs given to a

mother during labor is based on her weight, and it's an excessive amount for a baby to be subjected to.

We have to believe that birth is normal in order to begin to recover our confidence in the normalcy of our biological processes. But invasive medical interventions are routine. The baby in the womb, for example, is routinely bombarded with ultrasound, which is thought of as safe. But when I was growing up, X rays were thought of as harmless, not to mention DES and thalidomide. We rush quickly into new technologies, enamored of their newness, and often fail to appreciate that they may have unforeseen long-term effects.

Ultrasound is used routinely in pregnancy, in large part to determine information that a skillful practitioner can deduce by touching the mother's womb. But there's a study from the University of Dublin that shows that ultrasound actually changes cells, and that there was an increased incidence of left-handedness in babies exposed to it. That suggests that there is some effect from ultrasound that we aren't measuring, that we aren't taking into account. The American College of Obstetrics and Gynecology does not recommend routine ultrasound, reserving it for special circumstances, but we've created a climate of defensiveness in which physicians feel they must document all of their procedures during pregnancy and birth and must use all the newest available technology, otherwise they risk being accused of malpractice later on.

Most prenatal tests that women are exposed to are not necessary and are not supported by evidence. For example, women are routinely given blood sugar fasting tests during pregnancy. A pregnant woman is not supposed to go without food for that long, yet you have to fast to have these tests. The results include quite a few false positives. Those can be difficult to sort out, and are particularly difficult emotionally, because a false reading can put pregnant women into a worried and stressed state, the last thing they need.

Thirty percent of the births in the United States are surgical births, of which 22 percent are cesarean and the rest are forceps births and vacuum extraction. Electronic fetal monitoring is routinely used in births as well. This involves an electrode attached to the baby's head inside the womb. No test has ever shown an electronic fetal monitor to be any more effective or accurate than a simple stethoscope, but we've lost confidence in simple methods.

In fact, an experienced midwife can tell a lot just with her hands and ears. By turning birth into a stressful technological experience and by overusing drugs, we overpower the normal chemistry of birth, designed by nature to facilitate an ecstatic birth and to unlock a woman's dormant, instinctual maternal intelligence.

The good news is that despite all of these trends, the use of midwifery is increasing in the United States. In the 1970s, physician-attended births were 99.1 percent of total births. Now midwifery births stand at 8 percent nationally, and in New Mexico they're at 25 percent, the highest rate in the United States, because that state has had a licensed midwifery program since the 1970s. The appreciation of genuine evidence-based care is growing. There's an unprecedented coalition of U.S. birth organizations, the Coalition to Improve Maternity Services (CIMS), made up of groups that have come together to promote a ten-step program for mother-friendly childbirth, and there's a UNICEF "baby friendly hospital" initiative, which identifies ten steps to successful breast-feeding.

It's important that we learn about birth and believe in normal birth, and that we encourage women to seek births where they feel safe. I'm a supporter of home birth because I think it can be very empowering for women, but very few people realize that birth is safe in any setting, which is why most births in our country take place in hospitals.

Vaccinations are another potential source of toxicity and risk for children. We've covered the issue of vaccinations in *Mothering* magazine since 1979. Our roots were in the "back to the land" movement of the 1960s and early 1970s, when a lot of us wanted to create our own subculture and live a more natural life. As we began to have children, we had a lot of questions about birth, breast-feeding, vaccinations, and circumcision that we explored in the magazine. Historically, our coverage of the vaccination issue has always advocated informed consent and informed choice. More recently the issue has heated up, especially in relation to the question of mercury in vaccines.

Within hours of birth, a baby born in the United States is likely to receive a hepatitis B vaccine, the first genetically engineered vaccine. Hepatitis B, the disease, is mostly sexually transmitted. The theory is that somehow protection against this illness is going to last until children become teenagers or adults. The risk of hepatitis is a legitimate concern, but it is possible to test women for hepatitis B and then give the vaccination to the babies whose mothers test positive. But we don't do that. The public health approach in the United States is "get everybody when you can," and the "collateral damage" of a few bad reactions is considered acceptable. From the point of view of the parent of a child with a bad reaction, that's not acceptable at all. There are five times as many reactions to the vaccine as there are cases of actual hepatitis B in the childhood population.

At two months, infants are routinely vaccinated against several diseases. They can get up to nine vaccines at a time—diphtheria, pertussis, tetanus, hepatitis B, a strain of meningitis, and so on. Up until recently, all these vaccines contained a mercury preservative, thimerosal, that's been used since the 1930s. If an infant actually got these nine vaccines at one time, which is common at the two-month doctor's visit, the exposure to mercury could be 62.5 micrograms of ethyl mercury, 125 times the EPA guideline. And this standard was arrived at for ingested mercury such as one might eat in fish. There actually are no standards for injected mercury, so we don't know what a safe level of that might be. There is probably no really safe level. Europe eliminated mercury from vaccines in 1998, and in 2000, the United States began to get rid of it as well. But it was a phaseout, not a ban, so some children continued to get mercury-laden vaccines long after our public health officials discovered they were dangerous. There are also other potential toxins in vaccines, including metals such as aluminum, and no one is testing how these compounds might act synergistically.

There's also been a lot of controversy about increases in the rate of autism and whether those may be linked to certain vaccines. The rate of autism in the United States used to be about 1 in 2,000. In the last ten years, it's increased to 1 in 250. In the United Kingdom it's 1 in 85. Boys tend to be more susceptible. There's a chance that pregnant women's exposures to mercury via prenatal RhoGAM, dental amalgams, and other sources, as well as children's exposures to mercury in infancy, are at least partially to blame for this increase. Many parents whose children have developed autism strongly believe that it was caused by vaccinations because symptoms often manifested themselves so quickly after the vaccines were administered. The government and the vaccine manufacturers continue to deny any relationship, and the vaccine manufacturers have, successfully, pushed very hard for legislation to decrease their liability.

It costs $30,000 a year to care for an autistic child. The cost to fully vaccinate a child rose from $107 in 1987 to $367 in 1996. Vaccination revenues in the United States are now $1 billion a year, two times what they were in 1990, and pharmaceutical companies are among the only companies that are really making substantial profits at this time in our economy. So what should parents do? If you are inclined to vaccinate your children, ask for mercury-free vaccinations. It's fair to assume that most vaccines now are going to be mercury-free, but there are still pockets in the country where that's not yet the case. You can also ask for monovalent vaccines, which means one vaccine at a time, because there are some who feel the combination vaccines are riskier. If you are leaning against vaccinations, all the states have some medical exemptions, most have religious exemptions, and some have philosophical exemptions that you can explore.

Vaccines are very controversial, and all of us need to inform ourselves and to make our own decisions. There's a lot of information on the web on vaccinations, including a national organization called the National Vaccine Information Center in Vienna, Virginia, that puts out alerts on legislative action, and the entire transcript of the CDC's testimony at House hearings chaired by Congressman Dan Burton on vaccinations is available on the website of the House Committee on Government Reform (www.house.gov/reform).

Another very different threat to the well-being of children, but one that is just as alarming, is the aggressive intrusion of commercial media into the developing consciousness of children in their first seven years, which should be a time of innocence. A wide range of prominent psychologists and thinkers, from Jean Piaget to Rudolf Steiner to Joseph Chilton Pearce, have emphasized the crucial importance of these first seven years. As mammals we're designed to learn through play; that's how we develop the imagination that forms the basis for our later intelligence. It used to be that the time of childhood was sacrosanct, but now commercial interests are specifically targeting children, even toddlers, in a cradle-to-grave logo identification strategy. There are now four twenty-four-hour television channels for children, and there's aggressive, omnipresent advertising in public places. There's always advertising assaulting you, even in common space, that urges you to do something, to try to be something other than what you are.

It's very difficult to protect children from that. There's advertising, there are junk food vending machines, and there are televisions playing Channel One with commercials in schools. There are advertisements on nearly all clothing. Children have become little walking corporate billboards. Fortunately, there are a number of efforts afoot to challenge this state of affairs. One, called the Motherhood Project, issued a statement, "Watch Out for Children," that exposed commercial influences on children. Another group called Commercial Alert has issued a Parents' Bill of Rights that addresses these questions. So resistance is emerging.

This type of invasive commercialism is a form of violence to children. We also have to be aware that we too can be violent to our children in our own homes. I'm a product of the peace movements of the Vietnam War era, and I remember thinking at that time, "If I'm really interested in peace, I'd better make peace with my family first." I wasn't very peaceful with my parents, but I hoped I could change that and also raise peaceful children. Where does violence come from? How does it start? I don't accept that we're inherently violent. I believe that violence is learned in the first few years of life, when a lot of our behavior is imprinted. It's possible to change our habits and behavior later in life, but it's very hard because we're trying to overcome ingrained patterns we absorbed early in childhood.

It's during our first three to five years that we're supposed to learn trust, empathy, dependence, optimism, and conscience. Studies of psychopathic killers reveal that all had extreme disruptions in caretakers during the first three to five years of life. The availability of a consistent caregiver, someone you can depend on, someone you know is going to be there and loves you, is absolutely critical to normal development. It's imperative that we model nonviolence in the home, that we disarm our own inner environment. I urge parents to try discipline without punishment. Parents must, of course, be able to control their children's behavior at times, but there are many alternatives to punishment. It is possible to engage cooperation while still maintaining your authority. In a healthy family, the parents are leading, not dominating, and as their children get older, the parents change from being managers to being consultants in their children's lives.

I firmly believe the subtlest actions of everyday parenting can be the greatest tools for transforming the culture. If we extol the virtues of nonviolence in political situations, we must also find nonadversarial ways of relating to our children. It may seem easier in the moment to seize control, but domination is not healthy and does not really succeed in the long run. Many of us who have been parented by domination don't wind up being friends with our parents when we grow up, but we can break that pattern and make sure our own children imprint to love, not fear.

I am advocating that we regain respect for the inherent order of nature, our biological roots. Let's trust normal pregnancy and birth and the wisdom of our immune system. Let's protect the innocence of children and the common good. Let's disarm our inner environment. Healing the environment begins with our relationship to our own natures. If we can learn to stop suppressing what is natural in us, we will learn to trust ourselves and others, particularly our children.

Part V

Taking Action

Cycles of Continuous Creation

Katsi Cook

Katsi Cook's work spans many worlds. A wolf clan Mohawk from Akwesasne, Katsi is a mother of five and grandmother of three. Akwesasne, one of many member communities of the Six Nations Iroquois Confederacy, is located along the St. Lawrence River between northern New York and western Quebec and eastern Ontario.

Currently director and field coordinator of the Lewirokwas (yeh-wee-loh-gwas) Program (www.nativemidwifery.com) of Running Strong for American Indian Youth (www.indianyouth.org), Katsi comes from an enduring lineage of distinguished cultural and political activists, warriors, and healers. Her twenty-five-year vision of community- and culture-based aboriginal midwifery practice and culturally sensitive medical care has culminated in the establishment of the first free-standing birthing center in the province of Ontario, in a First Nations community at Six Nations, funded by the Ministry of Health of Ontario's Aboriginal Healing and Wellness Strategy.

In 1983, living and working within a mile of what would become identified as a National Priority List Superfund site at the General Motors Foundry adjacent to reservation lands, Katsi was confronted with questions from mothers in her care: Is it safe to breast-feed in an environment contaminated with PCBs and other organochlorines? Katsi's ensuing investigations led to Akwesasne's becoming the first community in the country to include human health research in the Superfund process.

❦   ❦   ❦

I COME TO YOU from the fireplace of the Kanienkehaka Mohawk people and from the current of the waters of life along the Kahniatarohwaneneh, the place where many waters converge, the mighty St. Lawrence River. I come to you from that place where I was born into the hands of my paternal grand-mother Kanatires, whose name, "She Leads the Village," continues to be handed down through the generations. From that place along the shores of the St. Lawrence River I come to you with a grateful heart.

I was born to Kawennaien (She Lays Down Her Voice), who came from an old Mohawk village, Kahnawake, located directly across the St. Lawrence River from Montreal, Quebec. When she was seven years old, my mother fell into the icy, rapid waters of the St. Lawrence in a sledding accident. In the days when antibiotics did not yet exist, the rheumatic fever she developed quickly consumed the mitral valve of her heart. Too delicate to attend school, she was educated at home by Catholic nuns. By the age of twelve, she spoke Mohawk, Latin, French, and English fluently. Her maternal uncle, the first Mohawk physician at Kahnawake, instructed her to spare her fragile health and never bear children.

I was her fourth child to be born at home.

Grandma delivered me at home in the big white iron bed in her farm-house bedroom in 1952. I was told that when I was born, my grandmother bundled me and placed me in a basket. Concerned about my mother's con-dition, it was another hour or so before she checked me again and found that I was bleeding from the umbilical cord stump. My grandma raised fifteen chil-dren of her own in the time of the Great Depression. Her colorful quilts were sewn from the worn clothing of her family, and she was an excellent seam-stress and needleworker. Using her common sense, she took a needle and thread and sewed up my belly button. Growing up in her care, my cousins and siblings would tease me: "You'd better not make Grandma mad or she'll take her thread back!" I used to sit in my little bed next to the big white iron bed she slept in, the bed where I was born, and search my belly button for that thread.

For these humble beginnings I am grateful, grateful I was born into the hands of my grandma. When I carried my first child at the age of twenty-three, I found my grandma's thread in the quickening that a new mother experiences. I found my path, my awakening, in the transformative power of birth.

In the Mohawk language, one word for midwife is *lewirokwas* (yeh-wee-loh-gwas). This word means "she's pulling the baby out of the water, out of the earth, or a dark, wet place." It is full of ecological context. We know from our traditional teachings that the waters of the earth and the waters of our bodies are the same water. The fluid that bathes the ripening flower of the ovarian follicle—the dew of the morning grass, the waters of the streams and rivers, and the currents of the oceans—all these waters respond to the pull of our Grandmother Moon. She calls them to rise and fall in her rhythm. Mother's milk forms from the bloodstream of the woman. The waters of our bloodstream and the waters of the earth are all the same water.

In the early years of my work at Akwesasne, I was confronted with one mother's question: Is it safe to breast-feed? In 1983, vast contamination of our local environment with industrial organochlorines—PCBs, most notably—was disclosed by the General Motors Foundry, which lay adjacent to the reservation territory. Earlier, in the 1970s, veterinary researcher Dr. Lennart Krook of Cornell University's College of Veterinary Medicine had revealed disabling fluorosis in local cattle as a result of atmospheric deposition of fluoride ash spewing from Reynold's Metals smokestacks on pasturelands on our reservation. Ensuing years would see the community's continuing struggle for remediation and restoration with an ever expanding circle of polluters and pollution sources throughout the Great Lakes Basin. If you look at a map of the world you can easily see that 25 percent of the earth's available freshwater is located in the Sweet Water Seas of the Great Lakes. We quickly realized that Akwesasne is a veritable sink of the Great Lakes Basin, down stream and down gradient from some of the world's most persistent and problematic pollution. On the way down the St. Lawrence River to the Atlantic Ocean, contaminated sludges and sediments bioaccumulate and biomagnify toxic contaminants in the food web of which we are all part.

At what would become the first National Priority List Superfund site in the country to include human health in its environmental assessments, Akwesasne emerged a leader in environmental justice practice, engaging community members, health care providers, and leading scientists and institutions. Fruitful partnerships have yielded great fruit in the improvement of our community's understanding and empowerment, sharing equity and authorship of scientific papers, with Mohawk women themselves as co-investigators in scientific research.

Women are the first environment. We are privileged to be the doorway to life. At the breast of women, the generations are nourished and sustained. From the bodies of women flows the relationship of those generations both to society and to the natural world. In this way is the earth our mother, the old people said. In this way, we as women are earth.

Science tells us that our nursing infants are at the top of the food chain. Industrial chemicals like PCBs, mirex, DDT, and HCBs dumped into the waters and soil move up through the food chain through plants, fish, and wildlife and into the bodies of human beings who eat them. These contaminants resist being broken down by the body, which stores them in our fat cells. The only known way to excrete large amounts of them is through pregnancy, where they cross the placenta, and during lactation, when they are moved out of storage in our fat cells and show up in our breast milk. In this way, each succeeding generation inherits a body burden of toxic contaminants from their mothers. In this way, we women are the landfill.

Realizing that mothers' milk contains an alphabet soup of toxic chemicals is discouraging stuff. Every woman on the planet has PCBs in her breast milk. Even in the circumpolar region of the north, our Inuit relatives of the Ungava Bay region of Nunavik have among the highest documented levels of breast milk PCBs in the world. Community leaders there state, "We will continue to do as we have always done" and consume an average of nine fish meals a month, primarily sea mammals like whale and seal. The essential fatty acids of this subsistence diet are highly protective of the cardio-vascular system.

At a Circumpolar Conference in the early 1980s, Inuit women expressed their opposition to a provincial evacuation policy for birth that was begun in the 1970s. Having been settled in villages by the government only since the 1950s, the Inuit had been accustomed to giving birth in igloos with assistance from community midwives. The evacuation policy obliged all women to give birth in distant cities to the south, separated from their families, their language, and their food customs. The cultural and social significance of birth to the strength of the social fabric and community health was removed. The Inuit midwives, among them Mina Tilugak, who was herself born in an igloo, say that "to bring birth back to the communities is to bring back life."

It is well established that the integration of valued lifeways and cultural acts like midwifery and breast-feeding into health care delivery systems is a fundamental step toward good health. In creating how we live we also create how we die. In a recent document from the Nunavik Regional Board of Health and Social Services to the Quebec minister of health and social services, the Inuit midwives say:

> There are few issues more fundamental to any people than birth. This intimate, integral part of our life was taken from us and replaced by a medical model that separated our families, stole the power of the birthing experience from our women, and weakened the health, strength and spirit of our communities. Over the last 20 years, how-ever, we have developed a midwifery system that has restored birth to our culture. Birth has come back to Nunavik, and with it, a sense of meaning and identity that can serve to rebuild the health of our communities.

"How do we teach the young about birth?" I asked my clan mothers in the longhouse.

"Begin with the story of the first birth," they said.

Our creation stories contain threads of worldview and relationship to the

universe that lie at the base of our belief systems and ceremonies. Creation stories are usually referred to as myth. It is said that myth is the accumulation of
a people's dreams. The Iroquois creation story tells of a chief's dream of a Sky
World inhabited by spirit beings. A celestial tree growing from the floor of
the Sky World was dying. The chief dreamed that the blossoms and fruits of
this sacred celestial tree were withering. He called for a dream-guessing feast.
A young woman whose name, Iotsitsisohn, means "mature flowers," traveled
to attend the feast, enduring tests along her path. Iotsitsisohn came into relationship with the chief and became heavy with child.

In my interpretation of the rich archetypal imagery, she leaned to gather
a yellow flower growing from the base of the tree to assist her in her puer-
perium. In doing this, she uprooted the sacred tree, creating a large hole in the
floor of the Sky World. Iotsitsisohn leaned deep into the hole to peer into the
vast blue expanse below. Seeds and bits of sacred things from the celestial tree
became embedded under her fingernails as she grasped the earth at the rim of
the hole, trying to break her fall. With the assistance of the winged ones, Iotsitsisohn, now Sky Woman, landed on the back of a great sea turtle. A muskrat
succeeded in bringing a clump of earth from the bottom of the ocean to put on
the turtle's back. Iotsitsisohn planted the seeds and bits of sacred things she
carried under her fingernails from the other world in this clump of earth. Danc-
ing in the direction the sun goes, she put into place the cycles of continuous
creation, continuous birth.

When her time came, she gave birth to a daughter, Katsitsioni, who followed her mother's ways upon the earth. Upon becoming a woman, Katsitsioni became pregnant by the turtle. She carried twin boys, who represent the
balance and harmony of life, the archetypal struggle between light and dark,
birth and death, integration and disintegration, good and evil. The evil twin
chose to be born from a hole he created in his mother's armpit with the flint
knife growing from his forehead. The good twin, born the usual way, spent
his days misunderstood by his grandmother and creating the earth as we know
it, in opposition to his evil brother.

From the severed head of Sky Woman's daughter, the mother of the cre-
ator twins, the moon was created, using tobacco, red willow, and ceremonial

fire. From her breast grow our life sustainers, corn, beans, and squash—the Three Sisters complex.

As human beings we have been given original instructions to follow in order to maintain the cycles of continuous creation and continuous birth put into place by Sky Woman and woven into being through the actions of her twin grandsons. This is the world we acknowledge in our continuing cycle of ceremonies, among them the thanksgiving to the maple tree in the spring, when we drink the maple waters for a cycle of days, perhaps fasting intermittently to prepare our blood, our bodies, and our spirits for the longer, warmer days ahead. And so on, through the cycle, we thank in turn the Thunder Beings, bless the seeds before planting, acknowledge the love of the sun for the earth expressed in the sweetness of strawberries, sing and dance for the corn, who taught us midwifery, and acknowledge and thank all that sustains life on this planet. Generation to generation, we continue these ways even in the midst of many oppressions. It is from these traditions that I declare the right of Mohawk women to discern for ourselves those things that come from our original mother and that we continue to hold as our own.

At each birth I have attended I have seen that new life falls from the hole in the Sky World of its mother's body. Embedded under its fingernails are the seeds and bits of sacred things that it will need and use in this life to fulfill its destiny. Like a dream, a fingerprint, a snowflake, each birth has its own interpretation, claims my teacher Roderico Teni, daykeeper of the Kekchi Maya.

Among the gifts of indigenous intelligence I use in my work with families is a knowledge of the Maya people of Guatemala—the Ways of the Days or the Tzolk'in. This family calendar is a sacred gestational calendar, an agricultural calendar that human beings use to relate to the spirit, the energy, or day-lord of each day in a cycle of twenty days that rotate in a corresponding number system, a count from one to thirteen. The spirit guardian of each day is related to a power of nature—wind, fire, sun—or a specific animal—dog/wolf, snake, jaguar, monkey, or bird—so that human beings can understand and relate to the energy of the day. Through this sacred count of the medicine of time itself, dreams, visions, ceremonies, and births can be interpreted. Our inner technology, our natural way of knowing, which is our intuition, can be awakened through the use of this sacred calendar. When Mohawks recite the Thanksgiving Address, for example, we express our love, appreciation, and relationship to the many elements of nature. The Maya further ask nature to move with us to create desired change. For example, ceremonies are held on certain days of the twenty-day cycle in order to gain their fullest efficacy toward the purpose of the prayer. In this workday world, ceremonies are commonly scheduled for the convenience of the participants. Even then it is possible to see the medicine of time at work in the interpretation and fulfillment of the ceremony over time.

There is a women's cycle as well as a set of days corresponding to male energy. Ajpu, the warrior day, and Imosh, also known as crazy day, represent men's intelligence, which can range from that of the protector in the battle for life to the unbalanced and violent. A person born in the women's cycle is likely to be a doctor or midwife or leader of some sort. The strongest connection for a healthy pregnancy and good birth can be made on the Kawok, the final and most concentrated day of the women's cycle.

In one young mother's prenatal dream, an unresolved fright/flight response from a traffic mishap, combined with public demands on the spiritual energy of her mother, in whose home she lived during her pregnancy, precipitated powerful dream imagery weeks before her due date. In her dream she was shut inside a two-room tent surrounded by black snakes. Peering through the opaque nylon mesh that separated the two rooms, she could see an older woman standing in the other room, handling the snakes. In her own space, the black snakes were thick around her feet.

"What did you feel at that moment?" I asked her.

"I was aware of the snakes but I was not afraid of them. I knew I wanted to get out of the tent," she said, "so I unzipped the zipper of the tent to get outside. When I stepped out of the tent, a huge white snake was reared up in front of me. I've never seen anything like it. It had a big head with white feathers coming down alongside its head."

Viscerally, intuitively, I sensed in the movement of her opening the zipper door of the tent both the cesarean section she would need to get her baby out safely and the big ceremony she would need to have done for her and her baby.

"When you doctor the mother, you doctor the baby," I learned from the Maya midwives.

In dreams, black snakes represent the problems of the people. The great white feathered snake of the woman's dream represented the archetypal white feathered serpent Cucumatz of the Maya people, known as Quetzalcoatl among the Aztec of Mexico. It augers powerful ceremony. There is a snake day in the Mayan calendar. The snake is the Mother of the Waters, both protector and justifier. Customarily our people are matrilineal and matrilocal. It is good practice to keep an expectant mother happy, contented, and away from fright. Sometimes her own mother is her best protector. Often you will see in traditional families that the expectant mother lives with her mother, or at least with her mother close by, reliving the "downfending" that Sky Woman's mother did for her as a young girl. The young Sky Woman was covered with cattail down and kept away from the petty concerns of the people who visited her family home, located far from heavily traveled trails. In the dream of the young mother, the old woman working with snakes reflected her mother's home, full of the myriad political and spiritual concerns of community people seeking her advice and ministrations.

I share these teachings of my mentor and brother Don Roderico Teni of the Kekchi Maya because we are concerned with the influence of time on our identities as indigenous people and on the knowledge we continue to hold, and the responsibility we have to maintain our lifeways for the benefit of future generations.

The duty of service to our people that each generation is given is an enduring message. The Mohawk way, *Onkwe honweh neha*, is a good way, the way of the people of the Flint. We continue to live. We're happy to be alive. We give thanks for the medicines.

Close your eyes in the place where you sit and draw oxygen from the room around you in long, deep breaths. Feel the current of your breath carry oxygen to the fireplace in each of the cells in your body. Use whatever image it is that you have in your own life, the experience of your own being that gives you strength, so that these things that you have been taught will be treated as prayers that you carry with you. You'll be able to use the higher thinking that human beings are capable of, so that your work will be strong, your road will be good, and you'll work with us in continuing to keep the cycles of continuous creation going ahead.

"In the night of the womb the spirit quickens into flesh," Black Elk said. In the darkness of this space I'm going to pull you babies out of a dark wet place. Each one of you has that youth inside you, to be strengthened to follow your road on this life, on this earth. You're strong if you use your best mind.

I give thanks, and pray that peacefully you will be born. I pray, hopefully, that peacefully your life will be ongoing, because it is that I think of you clearly, knowing you will always be loved. *Neh toh.*

Just a Little Too Well Behaved

Diane Wilson

For the past fifteen years, Diane Wilson has been fighting to end chemical warfare on the Texas Gulf Coast. Perpetrating this particular brand of bioterrorism are several of the world's giant chemical corporations, which have called her just about everything, including a terrorist. But sometimes we are best honored by who our opponents are.

The production of PVC plastics has ravaged the Texas Gulf Coast, Diane Wilson's ancestral backyard and fishing grounds and one of the richest and most diverse ecosystems in the world. The region's biggest PVC manufacturer, Formosa Plastics, is a multibillion-dollar global octopus that has systematically been plasticizing the Gulf with some of the most noxious poisons around. It's easy to see how Formosa got its reputation as the poster child for villainous corporations. This leader of Taiwan's petrochemical industry had environmental practices so appalling that 20,000 Taiwanese came out under threat of police violence to stop a proposed new $8 billion complex. That explains how Formosa ended up in Texas.

When the company announced its plans for a $1.3 billion expansion of a plant making the feed stocks for PVC, it expected the Lone Star State's customary confetti parade for creating jobs in an economically depressed region. But all that changed when Diane happened to read in the newspaper that her little Calhoun County, population 15,000, was rated in the nation's toxic top ten. She wondered if that might help explain the dolphins die-offs and alligators floating belly-up in her beloved Lavaca Bay. She decided to ask some questions and started holding meetings, and the rest is history, which in this case is her story.

It would be hard to make up a tale of mythic heroism more dramatic and colorful than Diane Wilson's true story of her epic battle with Formosa and other chem-

ical giants. This fourth-generation shrimper, the only woman shrimp boat operator on the Gulf and a mother of five, including an autistic son, is a larger-than-life, indomitable human being. Despite her lack of a college education and her dislike of chemistry, Diane taught herself to file successful legal briefs. Her knowledge of Formosa became so thorough that the company's lawyers routinely called her for information about their own outfit. After exhausting all legal means to stop the company's polluting, she resorted to civil disobedience and direct action.

The really amazing part is that Diane won, forcing Formosa and other companies to sign zero-discharge agreements. Though these commitments have yet to be fulfilled, Diane's victory highlights the viability of one of the most important strategies at our disposal: the adoption of zero-discharge technologies.

Renowned children's book author Molly Bangs published an animated children's book about Diane called Nobody Particular. Diane has been writing her own story, a book called An UnReasonable Woman. She got that right. But after all, look where reason has gotten us.

❀   ❀   ❀

I'M A COMMERCIAL FISHER from the Gulf Coast, from Seadrift, Texas. I've spent over forty years on the Texas Gulf Coast. I've fished the bays. I've been in the rivers, and I have watched those bays and those rivers systematically go down. In Texas and Louisiana, that's one thing we get to fight over: who's the most toxic state in the nation. Every once in a while Louisiana gets that honor and every once in a while Texas gets it. All the petrochemical plants come down the coastline, and they get tax abatements and cheap labor, and they use political corruption so they can get away with using those bays as a place to dump their waste. I think very few people have a sense of what it's like to live near the chemical plants down where I'm from in Texas and Louisiana. In the United States, there's a chemical explosion at a factory every hour.

At a Phillips 66 plant in Houston, an explosion a few years back killed thirty-two workers. At the Formosa Plastics facility near me, a huge, thick black fire burned for twenty-eight hours, and the company didn't even get a violation. Because I actually complain about these things, the *Houston Chronicle* did a story about me not too long ago which said that in my home town of Seadrift and in all of Calhoun County, I'm public enemy number one.

Bill Moyers did a documentary called *Trade Secrets* about PVC and the vinyl chloride industry that mainly concerned Louisiana, but Texas has quite a few vinyl chloride plants as well. Formosa Plastics is one of the biggest vinyl chloride plants. The occupational injuries and deaths associated with the work that the men in PVC plants do equal or exceed heart attacks and cancer as a cause of their mortality. The public does not know about it, and the media does not report it too much, unless you count Peter Montague's *Rachel's Environment and Health News*.

I have been an activist probably for about thirteen or fourteen years and I'm amazed that most people think that there are laws that protect us effectively, and a lot of folks even think these poor industries are being hamstrung and over-regulated. But thirty years after the passage of the 1972 Clean Water Act, which promised us the country's waters would once again be fishable and swimmable by 1982 and there would be zero emissions by 1985, a lot of our waters are as polluted as ever. According to the most recent government Toxic Release Inventory (TRI), 40 percent of our waterways are too polluted to fish or swim in, and 30 percent of our industries are in noncompliance. Those are just the ones that actually report it, so God only knows what's really going on out there. In the last ten years, there have been 30,000 closures of bays and waterways and over 250 million pounds a year of reported toxins going into our waterways. The Clean Water Act has failed miserably.

According to TRI data, in 1989 my county, Calhoun County, with a population of 15,000, was number one in the entire nation for toxic releases. By the following year, we weren't even on the list. Why? Our senators and the county commissioners, disturbed by the bad publicity, pressured to have a major toxic chemical delisted, and poof, the problem officially vanished. But those fifteen million pounds of toxic material are still sitting out there in the landfill. Formosa Plastics, one of the main chemical plants in my county that I have been fighting for a number of years, wasn't even on the list, though they were shipping millions of pounds of "distillation bottoms," toxic vinyl chloride residues, to Lake Charles, Louisiana, and burning them for heat. Why not? Well, Formosa said, "This is recycling, not waste release. We are recycling all these little dioxin-contaminated waste products."

I went and dug up a bunch of official files, and I found a number of letters from the state saying, "This isn't recycling. You need to report these numbers." They never did, and the matter seems to have been dropped. You have to learn to read between the numbers when you hear the EPA or industry talking about how "their numbers have come down." A company near me was always near the top of the toxic releases list, but is no longer on the list because it stopped dumping toxics into injection wells and started putting stuff in the Guadalupe River, which flows right down into San Antonio Bay, where we fish for a living. But for a technical reason that got that release off the list.

That was the reason I initially got involved in this environmental battle. One day I read in an Associated Press story that my county—they mentioned our county three times—was the number one county in the nation for toxic disposal. That just blew my mind. I knew there were chemical plants around, but I had never known the amount of what was going on. I am not a natural spokesperson. When I was a child, when people would come to the house, I would crawl under the bed to hide. But when I saw evidence of harm clearly in front of my eyes and people pretending it wasn't going on, I felt compelled to do something. So, I spent the next fifteen years fighting chemical plants and trying to keep the waste streams from contaminating our bays. When I first started, I didn't understand anything about chemicals or permits or TRI. I would call Union Carbide and Formosa and Alcoa and Dupont and BP Chemical and ask, "Could you kind of explain something about your numbers and where they come from?" It didn't work out too well.

Eventually, though, I learned how to find interesting material in official government files, and that's how I became such an expert on Formosa Plastics. They were starting the largest expansion of a petrochemical facility Texas had ever seen in our little bitty county, and nobody seemed to know anything about it. In our little old school district, they were eliminating seventeen teachers because we were in such bad shape, but Formosa had managed to get $200 million in tax abatements, and they immediately started building, bringing in 5,000 construction workers almost overnight. There had been no hearings; no information was available. In the beginning my only allies were poor divorced women; husbands of married women wouldn't let their wives get involved because it was too controversial. Since I'm a fisherman and my father was a fisherman and my brothers were fishermen and my cousins were fishermen, I tried to make allies with the fishermen, but the fisheries are in such crisis that most of the Anglo fishermen were very apathetic. They didn't believe you could fight city hall. As a matter of fact, they had lost so many battles that all they wanted to do was escape on their boats.

I'm actually a very mild, quiet person. But when I became aware of that TRI information, I went out and formed an environmental group. I called a meeting in my town and expected a few people, and I ended up with bank presidents and the chamber of commerce threatening me. I had senators down there in the fish house. I had people calling me a terrorist. They were certain, absolutely certain, that I was a spy for the state of Louisiana, because Texas and Louisiana were competing for the $2 billion Formosa Plastics chemical plant. There had been too much protest about its activities in Taiwan, which is why Formosa wanted to build in Texas or Louisiana.

So Wang Yung-chin, chairman of Formosa, was going back and forth between Louisiana and Texas and seeing which one was going to give him the most money for polluting their bays and waters. Texas got the prize because we gave him $200 million. And we gave him the little ship channels and we gave him banquets. Because I protested, I was considered a spy. I was considered a terrorist. Formosa threatened to sue me, and every single one of my board members quit because they were afraid that they were fixing to get sued.

People would come up to me very quietly and tell me they couldn't get involved because they had to have bank loans, and they had to have some of their kinfolk working at some of the plants. Because when the fishing industry goes down, you have a hard time. These are poor people, so sometimes during the winter when it really gets rough, they have to get jobs at these petrochemical plants.

But it's a myth to believe that you need a lot of people and a lot of money to resist, because you don't. All you need is commitment and belief. All it needs to start is you. All it takes is one person. I drew a line in the sand and decided they were not going to take those bays any longer. I had watched the dolphins die off. We had one of the largest dolphin die-offs ever recorded in the Mammal Stranding Network's history. All the dolphins, all the alligators—they were just sitting, rolling in the water. You would go out there and you would find hundreds of dead dolphins, acres of land with dead dolphins lying there, stretched out on the land.

We watched the red tides, the brown tides, the green tides. We watched Alcoa aluminum, with a permit from an agency, create a mercury Superfund site. Now you've got mercury in the sediment, mercury in the fish. And what do the shrimpers do? They sit on top of the Superfund site out in the bay, and they take the shrimp up, and folks out there are getting nice, mercury-laden shrimp.

I learned a very valuable lesson when I had a chance to go to Taiwan. My work had been covered by the underground Taiwanese press, and the Taiwan Environmental Union was holding demonstrations against Formosa Plastics and Chairman Wang because they had their own grievances with Formosa's behavior in Taiwan. A legislator named Chen invited me to come to Taiwan and talk to grassroots groups, unions, and others for two weeks. I learned of people being jailed, disappearing, being tortured and killed. That trip, those people, radicalized me. I felt like we, the people in the United States, didn't know how to make change. That lesson is best described by a quote from Henry David Thoreau. On his deathbed he is quoted as saying the only thing he regretted was that he was too well behaved.

So I've been working trying to enforce a policy of zero discharge for petrochemical plants on the Texas Gulf Coast. Zero-discharge law has been around for twenty years. It was in the Clean Water Act. It's a federal law and it hasn't been enforced because folks here are just a little too well behaved about asking for it and demanding it. But you can demand it, and anybody can do it; because if someone like me with a high school education who doesn't even like chemistry can get compliance from a petrochemical plant, then anybody out there can demand zero discharge at any type of facility they care to get invested in.

Ten years ago we could have demanded zero discharge, but nobody asked for it. When I first started this struggle I had never heard of zero discharge. I didn't even know it was possible. The only reason I found out about it is because I got a call from a businessman with a zero-discharge technology business in Houston asking me why I was fighting wastewater permits rather than just demanding the companies install zero-discharge technology. When I first brought it up, the companies claimed they had never heard of zero discharge. I spoke before a Gulf of Mexico symposium, and I was talking about zero discharge, and these CEOs were saying, "What are we talking about here? Philosophy?" It's not a philosophy; it's a technique. It can be done. There is a lot of available technology. It has been done for a long time. For instance, some Middle Eastern countries have been doing it, not because they were so worried about pollution, but because they had to conserve precious water. They couldn't waste their water. A lot of the zero-discharge technology arose from this desire to keep the water in a closed loop. That's one of its real benefits. You not only close the loop on pollution and avoid discharges going into the water, you actually save water.

Getting an agreement with Formosa took being outrageous, because in the beginning nobody believed me; they thought I was a real nut. Now they just think I'm a real persistent nut, but that's what it takes. I eventually had to go on three different hunger strikes to get my point across. One of them lasted thirty days. You'd be surprised what your body can do. It really can go for thirty days. You can go a long time, but I still could not turn the tide and get them to agree to zero discharge. By the third hunger strike, they admitted that there was such technology, but claimed that they just couldn't afford it. I wound up fighting their wastewater permit all the way up to an appellate judge in Washington, D.C.

There is something about being unpredictable—being unreasonable really worries them. I filed for every permit hearing. I lost my attorney, so I started filing my own briefs. I only have a high school education, and I'm not real logical or legal-minded, but I wrote my own briefs to the EPA.

So you can do a lot. A lot of it was just waiting for something to start materializing. I firmly believe there is a key to the universe. There is a universal law. If you put your commitment out there, I believe everyone is potentially miraculous—we could all be Gandhis. Sometimes things get so outrageous that you have to do something dangerous. You put yourself at risk, or your property at risk, and you can create miracles. You can create events. I've had people come up to me and want to know what immense organization was behind me, or who was directing me, and the scary thing was, there was nobody. It scared me at times. Because I kept thinking there's got to be somebody who knows what in the hell is going on and what I need to be doing. But there was nobody there. So you have to make the decisions, and they're hard decisions.

I don't believe in having a safety net when making these choices and taking these actions. They're scary decisions, and you always know you're on the path because you can smell your own fear, and you head straight for it. You have to head for the fear. Gandhi talked about soul power, and this is what it is. It comes from your soul. It comes from being on your path and realizing that there are things out there much bigger than yourself and what you think you've got.

I hadn't had much luck with the Anglo fishermen, so eventually I approached the Vietnamese fishermen. There had been a whole history of tension and hostility between the Anglo and Vietnamese fishing communities in Seadrift that got a lot of national attention about sixteen years ago. After the Vietnam War, a hundred Vietnamese families suddenly came into Seadrift, a real poor fishing town, and started crabbing. There had never been any attempt to facilitate communication, not by the entrepreneurs who had brought the Vietnamese or any of the state agencies or the Parks and Wildlife Department, which likes to regulate us, or any of the federal bureaucracies. When you've got a poor crabber who is trying to support his family and he sees another man put his crab traps too close to his, he gets upset about it. The Vietnamese didn't understand English and didn't understand the rules.

Words escalated into fights. There was a shooting, and then houses burned, boats burned. Then the Klan tried to come into Seadrift to march. Thank God we kicked them out of town, because they were very eager to seize the opportunity and make it a race issue. But these Vietnamese fishermen became the most dedicated demonstrators in support of my efforts. A *Houston Chronicle* reporter said the most surreal experience he'd ever had was to see Vietnamese fishermen protesting Taiwanese businessmen on the Texas Gulf Coast.

To make a very long story short, I did manage to stall Formosa's permit, but it was clear the EPA and the state had every intention of making sure they got their plant finished. When I realized how naïve I had been, that I could be right according to the letter of the law but still couldn't stop them from discharging, I was so outraged I decided to do the only thing I could think of that would shock people around Seadrift. I'm a very nonviolent person, so violence was out of the question. But I decided to take my own shrimp boat and sink it on top of their illegal discharge so that every time anybody went over the causeway, they were going to see that mast pole sticking up and they were going to think about Formosa's discharge.

Down on the Texas coast, your shrimp boat is real important. You can live in a shack. You can have a rusty truck, but by God, you've got to have a nice shrimp boat. For us, that's like a farmer with his farm. When I was fighting Formosa, I had been on those three hunger strikes trying to get them to zero discharge, to actually obey federal law. You run a traffic light and a cop's going to stop you, but Formosa was discharging into a bay system, and they didn't have their permit. They were violating the law. Absolutely no permit. I had an appeal going in Washington, and everybody knew it.

To really drive home to them how important this was, and to put things in perspective, that's when I took my shrimp boat. I had a forty-two-foot shrimp boat with a huge diesel engine. I had to have a winch truck pull out the engine because if I had sunk my boat with the diesel engine in it and gotten even a thimble of diesel fuel in that bay, they would have fined me royally and said I was the polluter. I had another shrimper with a boat sneak me out in the dead of night, pull my shrimp boat out there in the middle of a storm, and I was going to sink that thing square on top of Formosa's discharge point. They were going to have a monument to that discharge out there. But about two-thirds of the way out I had Coast Guard all over me. It turned out Formosa had hired, for $65,000 a year, one of my cousins, who had once been a fishermen's spokesperson, just to follow me around. He got wind of what I was about to do and told the Coast Guard. So, here it was at midnight in a storm and three Coast Guard cutters showed up looking for Ms. Wilson on her boat she's fixing to sink, and they accused me of "terrorism on the high seas."

They said I was facing nineteen years in the penitentiary and $500,000 in penalties. They confiscated the boat and tied it up to shore, but what I had tried to do finally woke the fishermen up. When they heard what had happened, all the fishermen—the Anglos, the Hispanics, and the Vietnamese—got out there in the middle of the bay on their boats and made such a stink that it caught the attention of the Associated Press, and it was all over the papers. Formosa finally got sick and tired of all the bad press, and they finally agreed to zero discharge.

So I got a zero-discharge agreement from Formosa Plastics. It took about five or six years to get. But about a month later I went to Alcoa, which had at that time the number one plant in the nation for toxic discharges. I went to them and said, "Now do we get a zero-discharge agreement or do we do the whole thing over?" In thirty minutes, they agreed to zero discharge.

I just want you all to believe, to know, that you can do it. Just believe in yourself and be outrageous. The author Molly Bang wrote a children's book about my story called *Nobody Particular*. That's a very appropriate title because, if there's one thing I want to get across, it's that if someone like me, naturally shy and with hardly any formal education, can take on some of the biggest companies in the world, anybody can do it.

Somebody said, "It's the reasonable woman that adapts herself to the world and it's the unreasonable woman that makes the world adapt to her." I'm telling all of you women to be unreasonable!

Why I Went to Jail to Protect
My Daughter from Toxic Polluters

Terri Swearingen

Terri Swearingen is a woman whose courage, dedication, and effectiveness have served as both model and inspiration for all those working for environmental justice.

She is a registered nurse, a mother, and a concerned citizen who took it upon herself to wage an extended battle against the siting and operation of the infamous WTI incinerator in East Liverpool, Ohio. This hazardous-waste disposal plant, the nation's largest, burns over 60,000 tons of toxic waste each year and spews out such toxic chemicals as mercury, lead, and dioxins.

Unbelievably, this incinerator was built 1,100 feet away from a local elementary school attended by over 400 children. Since the school sits on a bluff above the site, the incinerator's stack blows smoke directly onto the children each day. The WTI plant also sits in a floodplain on the banks of the Ohio River.

Starting in 1990, prior to the incinerator's construction, Terri began relentlessly researching, protesting, and organizing. She founded the Tri-State Environmental Council, a grassroots volunteer organization active in the affected areas of Ohio, West Virginia, and Pennsylvania. She testified before EPA and National Academy of Sciences panels, as well as before the Ohio State Medical Association and congressional committees. She has been arrested a dozen times for acts of civil disobedience, once inside the White House.

She waged outside-the-box media campaigns that caught the imagination of the nation. Using the media, she relentlessly held Al Gore's slippery feet to the fire to uphold his campaign and post-election promise to oppose the incinerator. Even so, the Clinton-Gore administration hit the ground backpedaling and permitted the WTI plant to commence operations. But Terri's efforts certainly caused them to pay a heavy political price.

175

Although she was unable to halt the WTI incinerator, Terri's perseverance led to a thorough national reappraisal of licensing requirements for toxic-waste incinerators. It's unlikely that such a siting could happen again, and no incinerator has been licensed since.

Terri has served on her county's board of health and on the board of the Environmental Background Information Center, which provides research and training to grassroots environmental justice activists. She is a current board member of Greenpeace USA. She has won countless awards and accolades from sources such as Time, E *magazine,* Mother Jones, *and the Presbyterian Church, as well as the most prestigious grassroots activism award, the Goldman Environmental Prize. In February 2003 she was presented with the first U.S. Public Interest Research Group John O'Connor Citizen Achievement Award.*

❀   ❀   ❀

I AM A REGISTERED NURSE, but my most important credential is that I am a mother. Although I'm not a scientist and I don't have a Ph.D., I do have a few letters following my name: N.M.B.S. Those are my credentials: No More Bull Shit.

I live with my family in the Ohio River Valley, where I've been involved in an effort to stop one of the world's largest commercial toxic-waste incinerators, run by Waste Technologies Industries (WTI). It's located in the floodplain on the banks of the Ohio River, in an impoverished, minority Appalachian river town. It's in a residential area where the closest home is only 320 feet away. WTI's smokestack is level with the front doors and windows of a 400-student elementary school that sits on a bluff above the site, 1,100 feet away.

While we haven't stopped WTI yet, we have been successful. Our efforts have halted other commercial incinerators from being built around the country. Because of our efforts, Ohio enacted a moratorium on the construction of new hazardous-waste incinerators across the state. We motivated Congress to conduct its first-ever hearings to look at the ways the EPA bent the rules to help the industries it's supposed to regulate. We prompted a nationwide freeze on construction of new toxic-waste incinerators and forced an overhaul of federal combustion regulations, including the development of more stringent limits for toxic heavy metals and a first-time emission limit for dioxin.

We compelled the federal government to acknowledge the serious risk that pollution poses to our food chain. More recently, citizens working to stop WTI have been credited as the driving force behind EPA's action to implement national siting standards for hazardous-waste management facilities. I'd like to share with you some of the strategies we used to achieve these successes and offer a vision for the future to prevent the continued poisoning of the planet.

I first learned about WTI in 1982. What caught my attention was that WTI was legally allowed to release 4.7 tons of lead into the air annually. Lead is a poison that is particularly harmful to the fragile developing brain and nervous systems of children. Any lead released into the environment is cause for concern, but when you consider that it will be raining down on children next door, that's criminal. In 1984, Ohio passed a law prohibiting the construction of any hazardous-waste management facility within 2,000 feet of any home, school, hospital, or prison, or within the floodplain. WTI was not built until 1991, seven years after that law was enacted.

A congressional hearing on WTI was held in 1992, and two major problems were identified. First, a site so close to homes and an elementary school poses an undue risk to an impoverished minority community. Second, WTI's permits are invalid, and rules were not followed. Top EPA officials admitted before Congress that they'd violated their own laws in issuing the permit, but they nonetheless allowed its continued operation. We've learned that the agencies set up to protect public health and the environment do so only if it's not threatening to any corporation.

It seems to be the government versus the people; multinationals versus the planet; and consultants versus common sense. People don't want these dangerous facilities, but the government does. Who's driving this process? Multinational corporations that generate too much waste, and the multinational waste

companies that want to profit from it. How do they get away with it? The ma-
chinery of government is directed against the people, not in the interests of
the people. Multinational corporations work against the interests of the planet;
they're only interested in profit. How do they get away with it? Incredibly
highly paid consultants versus common sense.

We show off the Statue of Liberty and talk about America as the greatest country in the world, but it's all about money. WTI puts American children at risk in violation of the law to promote the financial interests of the
money men behind the project. Money can make black white, round flat, dioxin
safe enough to eat on your cereal, and having an incinerator 1,100 feet from
an elementary school perfectly safe. It can buy politicians, regulators, lawyers,
and presidents.

But it isn't just a few people at the top who want to corrupt the system.
Evil doesn't occur because of one monstrous personality. One or two evil
people can corrupt a system only when there are hundreds of smaller faceless
players helping to carry out the agenda. Evil happens when good people ra-
tionalize fudging the truth. We must hold them all accountable. We must name
names.

Any time elected officials, regulatory agents, or industry employees are
responsible for a decision that allows the poisoning of our children, we should
put their pictures on a poster detailing their dirty work and distribute it everywhere so we all know who did it. We need to recapture America from the
corporate interests that run our government. If we don't demand accountability, we're going to lose our democracy.

It took a decade for us to learn that working only within the system didn't
benefit the people. We pursued legal, political, and economic strategies in our
efforts to protect our children, with little effect. That's when we engaged in a
direct-action campaign, which included peaceful, nonviolent civil disobedience. We broke the law to prevent our government from breaking the law.
We broke the law because we found the state of Ohio breaking its own law,
which was meant to protect citizens with a 2,000-foot buffer zone around dangerous facilities.

When our own government was not obeying the law, we had to break the law to draw their attention to the injustices. I've been arrested a dozen times, and I've spent many days in jail, including in Washington, D.C. Our first act of civil disobedience resulted in arrests. In 1991, following a rally attended by about 1,500 citizens, 33 people, including actor Martin Sheen, climbed the fence surrounding WTI. Of course we were arrested and thrown in jail. But it felt so good to go over that fence, to know that I was upholding a higher law, that I was working to protect our children. I was trying to uphold the law of human decency. I crossed the line because they crossed the line from a trust in people and democracy to a worship of technocracy and money. I crossed the line because they crossed the line between human values and human exploitation.

A week later we traveled three-and-a-half hours to the state capitol dressed in striped prison garb to issue "Wanted" posters for the real criminal: Ohio governor George Voinovich. The very bottom of the poster read, "Eyes blind to the facts, ears deaf to the calls of the citizens. If you see this man, do not try to 'comprehend' alone." When Governor Voinovich refused repeated attempts to meet with us and continued instead to defend WTI, we went to his mansion and posted "For Sale" signs on his lawn. We arrived at his home later than expected, catching him at home. As he jumped into a waiting car, we asked to speak to him, and his response was, "I have nothing to say." When reporters asked for comments, without thinking I just blurted out, "He's a weenie. He lacks the guts to face his constituents." To my embarrassment, the quote not only appeared in the next day's paper, but was highlighted.

So we decided to have fun with that. We used a hot dog to symbolize Governor Voinovich as "a weenie on waste." We had a weenie roast in front of his mansion, and I got to be the weenie governor. I dressed in a hot dog costume with a mask of the governor. I don't remember the exact words of my presentation, but it went something like this: "Frankly, I don't relish the pickle I'm in. I need to mustard the courage to ketchup with front-end solutions. I feel like a weenie, squeezed between a bun. it's no picnic being in this position. I think I'm going to get roasted."

We got a lot of media attention. We got our message out and we had fun doing it. We kept up the weenie campaign for about a year. In fact we never went to Columbus without delivering the governor a hot dog from the vendors outside. We had pressure-sensitive stickers made with the governor's phone number on a picture of a hot dog that said, "If you think the governor's a weenie on waste, call him." We went into all the grocery stores in Columbus and put those stickers on all the packages of buns and hot dogs. But one of the funniest weenie actions happened by accident. We heard that the governor was about to hold a press conference to announce his—get this— opposition to a toxic labeling law that would have required labeling for ingredients in products that cause birth defects and cancer. He was opposing it.

So we hid foot-long hot dogs under our coats and entered the press conference. When the governor took the podium, we pulled out our foot-long hot dogs and silently waved them in the air. The next day's newspaper headlines were hysterical: "Weenie-Wielding Women Whack Voinovich on Waste," "Wieners Cause Walk-Out," "Weenie Protesters Dog Voinovich." But the tactic was effective. The following month, Governor Voinovich announced a statewide moratorium on all new incinerators, which continues to this day.

Al Gore, in a post-election press release, pledged to stop WTI's operations. It was the very first environmental issue addressed by the new Clinton-Gore team. But after the inauguration, nothing happened. The Clinton-Gore team failed to keep its word.

In the spring of 1993 we participated in a month-long Greenpeace-sponsored bus tour of twenty-five toxic hot spots in eighteen states. The tour culminated in Washington, D.C., where we parked a mock incinerator, complete with a smokestack belching clouds of mock toxic emissions, right in front of the White House. We tied up traffic on Pennsylvania Avenue for over six hours until police, using jackhammers, could free us from the cement-filled incinerator.

We spent the night in jail, but the very next day, EPA chief Carol Browner announced an eighteen-month nationwide moratorium on hazardous-waste incinerators and a plan to overhaul and strengthen federal combustion policies. But WTI was exempted from the moratorium and is operating today. As our government continues to allow WTI to release daily emissions of dioxins, mercury, and lead, hundreds of schoolchildren spend their elementary school years breathing those vile by-products.

Our struggle is yet unfinished. We have to keep the pressure on until WTI is closed permanently. The laws and bureaucracies don't work unless we make them work. We have rights; unfortunately, we have to fight for them.

How do we prevent this problem of waste in the first place? Zero waste represents a global vision of sustainability. Zero waste is a way of bringing to reality people's desire to live on the planet in the way that nature intended, in a sustainable way, to live within the limits of the biosphere, not to dominate the biosphere. We have to look at the way nature exists. She has all her species living for millions and millions of years within this delicate biosphere. How does she do it? She constantly taps into the energy from the sun, and she doesn't make any waste. Zero waste. Nature recycles everything. So can we.

Not in My Front Yard,
or in Anyone's

Martha Arguello

MY WORK IS AT THE INTERSECTION of health, justice, and environmental concerns. I have been an organizer for the last twenty years in Los Angeles, and in the last three years I've been able to create opportunities, through Physicians for Social Responsibility (PSR), for physicians and public health folks to bring their expertise to communities engaged in front-line environmental justice struggles. But it's important to remember that while outside groups can play an important helping role, the movement for environmental justice involves communities speaking for themselves.

When I first started working with PSR three years ago, it was about the same time that the precautionary principle was becoming well known. The principle basically states that even in the absence of absolute scientific certainty, we have an ethical duty to act to prevent harm. For physicians, that concept is deeply rooted in the medical ethic to "do no harm." The second part of the principle states that affected parties have an absolute right to decide what an acceptable risk is, and what should and should not go into our communities. Until now, the burden of proof of harm has been on those who are affected by chemicals or industrial processes, but in the face of corporate science we are often left unable to prove with absolute certainty whether this cancer, this asthma, this rash, or this other ailment is directly linked to the chemical or the process we're being exposed to.

The precautionary principle says that we have a right to decide, we have a right to be at the table, and, given the limits of science, we still have an absolute moral obligation to act to prevent harm. In January of 2002, we organized the first-ever precautionary principle workshop in Los Angeles. We had over 110 people from different community groups, some working on pesticides in schools, some working to fight refineries, others fighting to clean up the former DDT plant that had been next door to them, and folks from Riverside fighting new truck stops and industrial parks. It was the most amazingly diverse group of people I've ever seen come together in Los Angeles around an environmental issue.

What was amazing about that day was to see what a ray of light the precautionary principle provides. It tells people, "You're not crazy for fighting, for knowing in your heart of hearts and in your gut that that power plant, that DDT plant, that benzene plant, or that refinery is what's making you sick." It completely validates our innate knowledge that says it is not okay to be putting toxic facilities or chemicals in my front yard or my backyard, or anyone else's. Folks who are involved in specific local environmental justice struggles often forget that there are many people all over the place fighting these types of battles. Many communities involved in environmental justice battles are communities of color that have never seen the environment as part of their struggle, and, in fact, as they fight that power plant or that mine, they still don't perceive of themselves as environmentalists.

To achieve real success we need to go beyond waging one isolated local struggle at a time. We need to be able to articulate a vision of the future. What does that future look like? How will we get our energy and our food? The precautionary principles is empowering: It gives you a strong philosophical basis for the idea that you have the authority and the right to decide what goes in your community. It is a great tool for us to begin to articulate a vision of what we do want.

A few months ago, the state of California finally began its process of developing environmental justice legislation, and that shift speaks to the increase in the power of this movement within the last ten years. Now California has a law that requires every division of the California EPA to have an environmental justice strategy and work plan.

Some of us went to the hearings and said, "We want you to implement the precautionary principle." It was fascinating to see the nervous faces of the regulators when we demanded that their decisions be based in ethics. We often ask ourselves, "How do they sleep at night?" Well, they could sleep at night because they had "risk assessment" to make them feel comfortable with their decisions, but the precautionary principle is a stick that gets poked at them and says, "No, your decisions are not ethical. Your decisions are hurting the health of our communities." That's not a comfortable place for regulators to be in, but it's important for them to remember that at one point they might have been very much like us and thought that they could change the world and make a difference. It can help tap into the desire that some of them must still have to bring real ethics back into their lives.

We've been figuring out ways to use the precautionary principle as an organizing tool. We've been able to push some of the California regulatory agencies toward more precautionary approaches. Those agencies that have been hounded at meetings by community members demanding public participation that moves beyond reacting and objecting, demanding that local people be situated at the very beginning of a decision-making process, do tend to change if the pressure keeps up. Now many different organizations are looking at the Los Angeles general plan and asking, "What does the city of Los Angeles say it wants to look like?" Environmental justice advocates are at that table saying, "This is what we want it to look like. We're going to zone out these toxic plants; we're going to plan them out of our communities."

I'm a member of the community pest-management team for the L.A. Unified School District (LAUSD), and we wrote one of the best integrative pest-management policies in the country. In the preamble of that policy is the precautionary principle. Community participation by parents, environmental and public health organizations, and other affected groups is built into how we will make decisions about how pests will be managed at LAUSD. We've been able to go from 134 chemicals that the district was using to 34. We have eliminated the use of most of the highly toxic pesticides. If it's a known reproductive toxin, it does not make the approved list. If it's a known carcinogen, it doesn't make the approved list. We meet once a month for three to four hours in highly contentious meetings, but it is community participation and action that determine how we will deal with specific problems. That may not sound like a big achievement, but when you realize the number of poor children who will no longer be exposed to whole series of toxic chemicals in their formative years, it was one of the biggest environmental justice victories in Southern California.

That use of the precautionary principle has been a real inspiration to other organizations and communities who are figuring out how to use it in their own battles. Public participation can just be a drain on activists' time and energy unless communities also have real power to make the decisions that affect their well-being. Some of the next steps forward will involve alliance building among poor communities, environmental groups, and green entrepreneurs who are producing clean, alternative energy and technologies, photovoltaics, and fuel cells. We can say, "We're all for economic development, but we want it clean, and we want it to be fair to our communities." We need to bring all these threads together, so that it's no longer about keeping stuff out of anybody's backyard, but about a vision of a truly healthy, clean, prosperous, sustainable way of life for everybody.

Globalizing Indigenous Resistance

Diana Ruiz

As the mining campaign coordinator for Project Underground, Diana Ruiz travels the world to expose the links between the devastating impacts of extractive industries and environmental racism, especially the exploitation of indigenous peoples. Most of the world's natural resources are in the South, often on the lands of indigenous peoples and people of color. It is a world that few in the North see or hear about, by design. If people knew about the jaw-dropping human rights violations and environmental devastation in these countries, they would be horrified.

Berkeley-based Project Underground is a unique and indispensable nonprofit organization dedicated to supporting communities that are resisting oil and mining industries and to challenging the abuses of extractive industries worldwide. Despite limited means, the group has played a decisive role in helping local groups organize effectively and coordinate with one another to resist the almost incomprehensibly destructive and rapacious behavior of corporations. Part of Project Underground's effort is to educate the world about the epic scale of this destruction, which Diana does with clarity, love, and strength. She has focused most recently on struggles in the western United States, Peru, and Indonesia, in places of critical biological as well as cultural habitat.

❧   ❧   ❧

VERY FEW PEOPLE ARE AWARE of the devastating environmental and social impact the gold mining industry has had on many indigenous communities around the world. But these communities are rising up and organizing against these powerful corporate polluters. I'm going to illustrate three separate struggles—in Nevada, Indonesia, and Peru—that focus on the Newmont Mining Corporation, the world's largest gold mining company, which is setting the standards for environmental and human rights violations here in the United States and abroad.

Historically, mining has been one of the most destructive of all industries, both socially and environmentally. In California alone, 120,000 indigenous people were wiped out at the beginning of the Gold Rush in 1848, and despite so-called technological advances, modern mining continues to be an extremely destructive industry in the United States and internationally, as photos of blown-off mountaintops and huge pits a mile wide and a half a mile deep readily show.

Gold has been primarily found on indigenous people's land. Some of these communities are among the poorest in the world. For over 500 years, mining interests have targeted these communities because they are politically marginalized and isolated. The first phase in the process of extracting gold is getting access to land, by offering to buy it at an extremely low price or just expropriating it. Recently companies have been getting less crude and more cunning in that they now offer gifts, bribes, and menial short-term jobs for the often traditional tribal people whose land they covet. They then force them into a wage economy and use divide and conquer tactics to weaken their communities.

Once the company has access to the land, the production process begins. This usually entails using dynamite to blow off the top of a mountain, extracting huge amounts of rock, and then using cyanide to leach the trace amounts of gold from the rock. Before 1960, mercury was the chemical of choice for these companies. Both cyanide and mercury are powerful neuro-toxins. The companies use sprinklers to spray a cyanide solution that also contains ammonia over heaps of crushed rock, twenty-four hours a day, so that the specks of gold can be slowly dissolved and released from the bottom of the rock pile. This very unsafe process is being used at a growing pace in more and more places. In some countries such as Indonesia, where there is a lot of rainfall, the pools of cyanide solution left on the leaching pads run off into streams. There are no containment units or water treatment facilities whatsoever.

Gold mining also opens up huge amounts of rock to erosion. The exposure of usually buried minerals to air and water creates a chemical reaction that produces sulfuric acid, known as acid mine drainage. This solution releases heavy toxic metals that are known carcinogens into the water. People in downstream communities very quickly start developing skin rashes, and fish start dying. In poor countries, these communities use these waters not only to bathe, but as their only drinking water. Acid mine drainage actually continues to get worse long after a mine closes. The larger the amount of rock exposed, the higher the levels of subsequent acid drainage. Eventually the groundwater is totally poisoned and all aquatic life in nearby streams and rivers is completely destroyed.

The next biggest problem with this industry, after cyanide, mercury, and sulfuric acid toxicity, is the problem of waste disposal. In the United States, an average gold mine produces three million tons of waste for one ton of gold. In some other parts of the world, the industry actually dumps these wastes right into the ocean. In Nevada, in 2000 alone, Newmont Mining dumped 220 million pounds of toxic chemicals right into nearby streams, contaminating the groundwater. Newmont owns nine of the largest mines in the state and has reported the bulk of toxic releases for the state. Newmont's operations are on Western Shoshone land. The Western Shoshones signed a treaty to share their land with the U.S. government in 1863, but our government failed to honor the treaty and now sells and leases the land's mining interests. Nevada has been ranked one of the top five most toxic states, and Newmont is one of the largest polluters in the United States.

Here in the United States, we have the Environmental Protection Agency and other agencies that supposedly help regulate these industries. They're not doing their job very well, but these companies are also going abroad, where there are no environmental protection agencies at all. Newmont has two operations in Indonesia, one in Sulawesi and one in Sumbawa. Newmont representatives met with the Indonesian government and with the community of Sulawesi and said they were going to use the safest technology possible and manage the waste by using a technology called submarine tailings disposal. Basically that means they dump mine waste right into the ocean. They use pipes that run from the upland facilities all the way down to the ocean and dump all the waste rock, the mud, and the toxic chemicals right down to the seabed, a process that would be totally illegal in the United States and in Canada. Of course, scientists have found high levels of biaccumulative carcinogenic chemicals in the bay. Newmont is actually about to shut down one of its Indonesian operations. It has no plans to clean up the six enormous open pits that have been left behind, and it claims that the two thousand tons of mine waste that it dumped into the ocean every day for six years will just naturally disappear in a few years.

In Peru, mining's destructive and violent legacy dates back all the way to the 1500s, the beginning of the bloody reign of the conquistadors. Today it is facilitated by institutions such as the World Bank and the International Monetary Fund, which pressure developing countries like Peru to rely on selling their natural resources in the world market. The Yanacocha gold mine, Newmont's largest, has done nothing to improve the well-being of the province of Cajamarca, the second poorest province of twenty-four in Peru. Lands have been destroyed, water and soil serverely contaminated, and communities disempowered.

But the good news is that around the world, communities are rising up and organizing themselves locally, regionally, and globally to defend their human rights, their right to clean air, clean water, self-determination, and autonomy. In 1999, the first-ever People's Gold Summit was held, with community representatives from twenty-one countries. At the end of the summit, the representatives wrote a declaration demanding an end to toxic-based open-pit gold mining, to ocean dumping, and to military, paramilitary, and mercenary activity used to secure the mines. One company emerged as the biggest villain, and that was Newmont. These indigenous people in some cases wanted mining to stop entirely, but they were demanding cleanup and proper compensation in all mining operations.

After that conference, a lot of the communities in Southeast Asia felt that there was a need to have a conference on submarine tailings disposal, because no one seemed to have adequate information about the repercussions of that technique. So in April of 2000, the first-ever Submarine Tailings Disposal Conference took place near Sulawesi, where the Minahasa Raya mine is located. Activists and scientists from the United Kingdom, Australia, the United States, and Southeast Asia, as well as community representatives, met to compare notes about submarine tailings disposal and its disastrous impact on human health in coastal communities and on the fishing economy. After the conference they went to Jakarta and requested a meeting with the minister of the environment. The people from Buyat Bay and from Sumbawa were able to state their case: They wanted Indonesia to stop issuing permits for submarine tailings disposal by gold mining companies. The minister of the environment had heard that there had been protests in these islands but hadn't paid much attention to them until international activists and scientists showed up and explained the health and economic impacts of this disposal method. He agreed a day later to stop issuing permits for the use of submarine tailings disposal and to suspend Newmont's permits. A month later, this minister was dismissed, with no reason given, but the communities in Indonesia are determined and feel strongly that they can win this struggle.

Another even bigger international meeting took place in 2002 in Bali, in advance of the World Summit on Sustainable Development. Eighty-five people came together from twelve countries to talk about the impacts of gold mining, including submarine tailings disposal. There were a number of outcomes: a demand for a mining moratorium, a "Women in Mining" statement, and a declaration by the Southeast Asian communities affected by mining.

In Peru in 1999, 10,000 rural, urban, and indigenous people marched in the streets of Cajamarca to stop the expansion of the Yanacocha mine onto

Mount Quilish, a site sacred to many local people and the only natural drinking water source for 15,000 people in Cajamarca. A year later, these communities won the battle to protect Mount Quilish, and the municipality declared it a conservation area. Newmont is appealing this ordinance in the Peruvian supreme court, but the community is even more united now. Urban and indigenous groups have organized huge joint protests in Cajamarca to pressure candidates in the upcoming national elections to resist Newmont.

Around the world, communities are starting to succeed in challenging the mining industry and holding corporations accountable. It is a slow process, but it is happening.

Here is an excerpt of the statement on women and mining that came out of the Bali Mining Workshop. It gives a good sense of the rising resolve and awareness of this global movement.

We, the 74 representatives of communities affected by mining, nongovernmental organizations and activists from 15 countries of Africa, Asia-Pacific, Latin America, Europe and North America, have gathered in Bali from the 24th to the 27th of May 2002, to tally the impacts of the global mining industry on our communities and ecosystems, and to assert at the occasion of the World Summit for Sustainable Development that mining as we know it today is unsustainable and runs counter to people-oriented development.

Women are among the worst affected by mining in their various countries. Therefore, it is important to look at the entire mining industry from the perspective of a woman, from the experiences of women miners, from the women in communities affected by mining. We assert the following: Mining is completely unsustainable for us women, and offers no viable opportunities, social or economic. We believe that there are widespread negative impacts on women's lives in all mining regions of the world. We also believe that mining industries have no remedial solutions, nor mitigative or preventative measures for the human rights abuses and atrocities on women who work in mines or live in mining affected communities. Therefore, we oppose the entry of any new mining projects, or expansion of existing mining projects, especially in indigenous regions.

We want to practice our traditional livelihood systems based on land and forest. We want economic and social progress, which enhances the conservation of these resources as opposed to making for their destruction. And as mining destroys our land and forests, we demand the continuation of our traditional livelihoods and the creative pursuit for alternatives to mining. We demand legitimate entitlements for women with regard to land and natural resources. Where mining exists or must continue, we demand equal opportunity for women in the mining sector. We demand wages and working conditions for women miners which strictly follow international standards and ensure equality and equity without discrimination based on gender. We demand the abolition of child labor in all mines. We demand a gender audit of all mining projects.

Overcoming Environmental Racism

Henry Clark

Henry Clark is a legendary figure, one of the most effective and well known organizers working for environmental justice in Northern California, or anywhere in the United States, for that matter. His base is the Bay Area's Richmond district, a largely low-income and minority community notorious as a nexus of toxic industrial pollution and social neglect.

As executive director of the West County Toxics Coalition, Henry deals day to day with the severe negative health impacts of petrochemical company facilities and their noxious pollutants. Richmond has been the site of some of the Bay Area's most spectacular industrial accidents, and Henry and his organization's astonishing and hard-won successes have become models for many other disenfranchised communities here and abroad as they struggle to defend their human rights and protect themselves against the poisoning of their air and water.

Henry brings an astute strategic sense to what he recognizes as a long-term struggle. He has carefully chosen his battles, patiently organized communities, and built essential bridges into the entrenched power structure. His unbending refusal to see Richmond continue to be used as a dumping ground has brought a series of surprising victories that show just how great a difference one person and one community can make. Henry knows that resistance furthers.

❀   ❀   ❀

I'M WITH THE WEST COUNTY TOXICS COALITION (WCTC),
based in Richmond, California. The WCTC was started in September of 1986
so that residents of the Richmond/West County area could fight back against
the chemical assault that we were experiencing, primarily from the Chevron
refinery in Richmond, the largest oil refinery in the western United States.
Several other chemical companies, such as the General Chemical Company,
are also located in Richmond, and there are numerous hazardous-waste facilities as well. But by and large, Chevron is the major operation that has had
the most serious problems over the years, including periodic fires and explo-
sions and numerous accidents, such as the infamous 1989 explosion and fire
that sent black clouds of toxic smoke over the entire region for a week.

On July 26, 1993, there was a massive sulfuric acid release from General
Chemical, a company that refines sulfuric acid that it gets from the Chevron
refinery into electronic-grade sulfuric acid. The North Richmond area was en-
gulfed in a sulfuric acid cloud and over 20,000 people went to local hospitals. The company was fined about $1.8 million by the Contra Costa County
district attorney's office rather than face criminal charges. It did not have a
permit to be engaged in the type of loading and unloading operation that resulted in the release. WCTC advocated that the fine money come back to the
community rather than go to the regulatory agency, from which we see little or no benefit. That fine money ultimately went toward building a health
center in the North Richmond community, a low-income, primarily Afro-
American community that's on the front line of the chemical assault. That
center is built now and has been in operation for about a year, providing general medical services to the community as well as environmental health education, and because of the role the WCTC played in advocating for that
health center and making it happen, we now have a permanent seat on the
board of directors of the North Richmond Center for Health. Presently, I serve
as chairman of the board.

I want to give you a few other examples of the types of problems we face and our organizing efforts. There's a hazardous-waste incinerator at the Chevron Arco Chemical Company in North Richmond. The Chevron Arco Chemical Company is the pesticide division of Chevron. This incinerator has been in existence since 1967 on a so-called temporary permit. Going back to 1990, Chevron had been trying to get a permit to expand the amount of waste that it was burning in the incinerator from approximately 80,000 tons to up to 120,000 tons a year. We opposed the expansion of the incinerator. We organized a postcard-writing campaign among the residents in the surrounding communities. We collected about 1,200 signed postcards that we and some community leaders took to the Department of Toxic Substance Control office in Berkeley, one of the lead agencies on the project, and we expressed our dissatisfaction with Chevron's request for a permanent permit to expand the waste incinerator.

About two weeks later we received word that Chevron was withdrawing its application to get a permit and, in fact, the incinerator was going to be closing. That was the result of a couple of things: not only our organizing of residents to oppose the expansion of the incinerator, but also Chevron's desire to get out of the chemical production business and focus on the refinement of oil. So, for a combination of reasons, the incinerator was closed. That eliminated a major source of chemical poisons that residents were exposed to in the area.

I was part of a delegation that went to Nigeria last year to explore how U.S.-based oil companies operate there. Chevron has operations in the Niger Delta area, as do Shell and the French company Total. The companies here in the United States pay lip service to wanting to be good neighbors and talk about environmental protection, but when you leave the United States (and it's bad enough here), when you go to countries like Nigeria or South Africa, you see that they can recklessly destroy the environment there with impunity. They dump garbage in streams that people use for their livelihood. Oil is being taken out of their yards, but the oil companies do not invest in the community at all. They do not hire local people. They say that since they cut a deal with the Nigerian government whereby it gets about 60 percent of the take and the oil companies get 40 percent, it's the Nigerian government that should be investing in local communities. But the government there is corrupt, and the people cannot depend on it to invest anything in their communities. When villagers complain or demonstrate, the oil companies call in the police and the military.

Because of our longtime involvement in environmental justice issues here at home, we have formed connections with communities internationally that are facing similar problems and issues but are not as experienced as we are.

We have waged some long, hard struggles but there have been many victories. For instance, there was no early warning system in Contra Costa County when we first started. When there was a chemical release or an explosion, we would learn about it on the ten o'clock news or read about it in the newspaper the next day. We advocated for an early warning system to alert residents when there was some chemical disaster. At first elected officials and industry people didn't want to hear anything about a warning system being put in place, because if you have a warning system, that's alerting residents to the fact that there's potential danger around, and they didn't want people to have that conscious awareness. Finally, after numerous chemical disasters, they got the message, and now Contra Costa County has an early warning system in place. If there's any kind of a chemical disaster or an emergency that people need to be aware of, they'll receive a recorded message by phone indicating the nature of the release, and all the sirens will go off in the affected area.

I'm now a member of the Contra Costa Hazardous Materials Commission, where I can talk about environmental justice and the disproportionate impact on our communities. There's a study that we were part of called "Richmond at Risk." It looked at the twenty largest industrial operations in the city of Richmond and the socioeconomic characteristics of the community, and in every case it showed that those industrial operations were located in and around communities of color where 70 to 75 percent of the population was Afro-American and 20 to 25 percent of the population lived below the poverty line. That's what we call environmental injustice or environmental racism, because we don't think, by any stretch of the imagination, that these chemical companies just happened to be located in low-income communities of color. That's the situation we're fighting. We've been working on getting Contra Costa County to incorporate environmental justice policies in its planning process.

The key to achieving environmental justice is that communities have to organize themselves. None of these victories would ever have occurred if our communities were not organized to hold these companies and these agencies accountable to work toward a clean, green, safe environment for all of us.

The Global Politics of Precaution

Sharyle Patton

Sharyle Patton has an exemplary history as an international environmental, social justice, and women's rights activist. She is perhaps most visible for her work as codirector of Commonweal's Health and Environment Program, where with her husband, Michael Lerner, she has developed key programs that focus on three critical areas: cancer, children at risk, and environmental health. But she has also waded into the tar pits of global treaty negotiations, where her unbreakable perseverance and patience have brought a high social profit for both people and the environment.

As the northern co-chair of the International Persistent Organic Pollutants (POPs) network, she has helped link over 300 public-interest groups around the world that are active in United Nations negotiations dealing with chemical contamination. Thanks in large part to that work, ninety governments signed a landmark 2001 UN treaty that will ban some of the most dangerous chemicals and severely restrict the use of others. She remains deeply involved in this network, currently serving as co-chair of its Community Monitoring Working Group, through which she helped organize a grassroots U.S. campaign to influence the federal government's retrograde position at the 2001 treaty negotiations. She also works extensively on the international stage to support the efforts of NGOs and civil society to educate governments and leaders about the importance of creating a POPs treaty strong enough to be genuinely protective of human health.

Sharyle served as director of the Citizens' Network for Sustainable Development, a national network that grew out of the United Nations' 1992 Rio Conference on the Environment and Development (UNCED). She has been a civil society representative on delegations to a large number of major UN world conclaves, including the Cairo and Beijing women's summits.

Sharyle is the coeditor, with Alexandra Rome, of "The People's Treaties from the Earth Summit" (Commonweal, 1993), an annotated compilation of the treaties negotiated by NGOs from around the world in Rio. This tireless organizer has also somehow found the time to be a highly accomplished videographer who over the past twenty years has produced a large body of work, including the PBS NOVA docu-mentary The Man behind the Bomb, *the story of peace activist and nuclear physi-cist Leo Szilard.*

＊　＊　＊

SANDRA STEINGRABER IS A BIOLOGIST, writer, and poet who talks about environmental health. Her newest book, *Having Faith*, tells the story of her pregnancy, the birth of her daughter Faith, and her breast-feeding ex-perience. She describes the terrible dilemma of being a breast-feeding biologist who knows the great harm chemicals now found throughout the environment and in breast milk can sometimes have on a developing fetus and an infant. Sandra Steingraber is now breast-feeding her six-week-old son Elijah and con-tinues to breast-feed the now two-year-old Faith. It's quite inspiring; she's a poster person for breast-feeding.

She knows that although there are potentially harmful chemicals in breast milk—it is in fact the most contaminated food on the planet—breast milk re-mains the best food for a baby, unparalleled in its benefits to the developing immune system. Breast-feeding is also psychologically crucial, providing a baby's first experience of learning to trust the universe. A child learns at its mother's breast that there is a place in the universe of comfort and connection. The fact that breast milk is contaminated and that mothers are conflicted about it is absolutely outrageous.

The fact that contaminants are found in breast milk is an indication that there are toxic chemicals to be found in all our bodies. Measuring chemicals in breast milk is one way of testing for the presence of chemicals, because breast milk is produced by using stored fat in a woman's body, fat that can store dozens of toxic chemicals. And of course all our bodies contain fat, and this fat is the perfect residence for many toxic chemicals.

If you think you're safe because you live in the woods, off the grid, eating organic food and wearing organic cotton clothing, let met tell you about my husband, Michael Lerner, and me. We live in Bolinas, California, in a rural, beautiful place on the coast. We eat organic food and are careful about the products we use. We breathe some of the freshest air that's left on the face of the earth. Recently we had our chemical body burden tested in a pilot study conducted by the Mount Sinai School of Medicine, the Environmental Working Group, and Commonweal. We were tested in the same group as Bill Moyers for his recent documentary about the chemical industry, *Behind Closed Doors*. We were monitored for about 210 chemicals, including organophosphates, organochlorines, and heavy metals. The levels in our blood and urine were pretty much similar to those of our colleagues who live in Boston and New York. My own levels of dioxin and PCBs are right up there with those of my friends who live in "cancer alley" in Louisiana. So these problems of environmental toxicity cannot be solved by individuals' changing lifestyles, although personal decisions about what you eat and what products you use can help somewhat and do send a message to manufacturers about their products.

But because many chemicals have the capacity to travel thousands of miles from where they are produced or used, due to their particular chemical characteristics, toxic chemicals need to be regulated at the international level. For example, dioxin produced in Iowa finds its way up to northern Alaska. The PCBs found in soil sediments on the shores of Cameroon, which has never used or produced these chemicals, could come from many different sources. So wherever we live, we are all exposed to hundreds of chemicals, a veritable chemical soup. Only legally binding global decisions that address global exposures will truly protect human and ecosystem health. The United Nations has taken on this chore of global regulation, beginning with twelve chemicals and a process to assess more.

The UN may seem to be merely a group of diplomats continually producing turgid documents devoted to stating the unexceptionally obvious in the most complicated manner possible, but let me give you another impression of the UN, from my own experience of lobbying there on behalf of the International Persistent Organic Pollutants (POPs) Elimination Network. There are elements of the UN negotiating process that look like the legendary hero's journey, and let me explain why I use this metaphor. In each case, the vision-quest traveler leaves ordinary activities behind and engages in a long journey requiring particular clothes, special structures, perhaps particular rituals, and sometimes a consciousness aimed at other than everyday thoughts. During UN negotiations, diplomats all over the world are hopping onto planes and going to a faraway location, to some special building dedicated to decision making, which they enter often weary and jet-lagged. The climate in these buildings is always the same, adjusted for people wearing light wool suits; whether it's Bangkok or Canada, it's always the same temperature. All the people at the meeting have really stepped out of their ordinary lives to think about these things, and negotiations go on night and day for quite some time. When we reach the point where the UN budget says, "Okay, negotiations have to stop," the clock is stopped at midnight, but we continue negotiating until the wee hours of the next morning, and perhaps well into the next day. We really are living outside of our ordinary lives and outside of time.

Sometimes the frivolous ideas fall away and the best thinking emerges. It's a transformative process. At the end of deliberations, tears are streaming down the faces of some of the delegates. There's been some kind of big change, and what we have produced is a liturgy on which we will base action and decisions, and which we'll work to interpret for years to come. The quest for a new vision is often successful, and some of these staid, determined diplomats can be considered heroes.

The UN can, at times, be a dynamic, flexible organization, and when it comes to thinking about chemicals, there really has been a valuable process, and much progress. Part of that progress has happened because of nongovernmental organizations interacting with UN diplomats. When the first earth summit took place in Rio in 1992, most of the NGOs were kept far away from the actual negotiations, but since that time NGOs have gotten more access to the UN process. We're starting to be able to talk to more delegates during the negotiations themselves, and at this point, some governments actually seek out NGOs for our expertise, for the studies we have done and for the alternatives we can offer. It was Sandra Steingraber's presentation to government delegates at one of the negotiations about chemicals in breast milk that really helped channel the direction of government discussions about prevention and precaution. Delegates also look to their domestic NGOs for evidence of political will within their own countries, as a guide to setting new priorities. It's important to understand that the UN is accessible to NGOs that have an area of interest. If you're a serious group interested in chemicals, you can go to the UN and continue to help the delegates hammer out the implementation of what we're calling the POPs Treaty—the Persistent Organic Pollutants Treaty, now called the Stockholm Convention because it was signed in Stockholm in May 2002.

Even before the Stockholm Convention enters into force, UNEP—the United Nations Environmental Program—is organizing workshops around the world to get the treaty implemented. Countries and NGOs around the world are involved in implementing the treaty. You can get involved too.

These UN treaties can be very useful to us in advancing the precautionary principle. The precautionary principle is the most important guiding idea we have to help us in the urgent task of dealing with new technologies and reevaluating old ones. It means, basically, "better safe than sorry," and "look before you leap"—it's really common sense. But common sense is not what our society has used in dealing with chemicals. There are about 80,000 chemicals registered for use. Of those, less than 10 percent of the industrial chemicals produced in large quantities, which means over one million pounds per year, have had a full complement of basic toxicological screening. There is no data at all for about 40 percent. Nobody has a clue what these chemicals can do to us. There's more data on the health effects of pesticides, but information about their reproductive and developmental effects is often lacking.

Most of these chemicals were unknown before World War II. In our bodies, all of us, wherever we live, harbor detectable levels of about 200 of these new chemicals. We know that there are some novel chemicals created by by-products of certain industrial processes that we don't yet have any procedures to identify or measure, so we may be carrying as many as 600 new chemicals, according to an EPA report. Nobody knows the long-term effects of many of these chemicals, either singly or in combination, or how they may affect particularly vulnerable populations, like children, the elderly, or the developing fetus.

Originally, diplomats around the world wanted to have a global summit on toxic chemicals to take on the whole issue. The United States and some other countries said, "If we do that, it will just be a talkfest and we won't get anything done, so let's start someplace where we can all agree, and then we'll build from that success. Let's do a smaller conference on persistent organic substances, chemicals that tend to stick around for a while, where there's some kind of definitive cause for concern." So they selected a short list of twelve chemicals that everybody agreed were bad actors. This list includes nine pesticides, including DDT, some PCBs, and some dioxins. A lot of countries had already banned some of the pesticides. The idea was to help countries implement their own laws and figure out how to get rid of stockpiles, clean up reservoirs, and destroy these chemicals in a responsible way.

Everyone had agreed for at least twenty years that these chemicals were bad, but what NGOs brought to these negotiations was the fact that many of these chemicals were also endocrine disrupters, that is, substances that the human body erroneously recognizes as hormones or as triggers for cascades of events within the body. When such triggers mistakenly direct the way the growing body develops its immune, reproductive, or neurological systems, damage can occur. If you have one such chemical in your system and you're a pregnant woman, the body might allow it to shoot right across the placental barrier and change what your baby is going to be like, how its immune system is going to function, how it's going to think, and how its motor responses are going to work.

At the UN, nongovernmental organizations spent a lot of time teaching delegates about endocrine disrupters. These chemicals are harmful at really small levels, and timing is critical. It's not just how much of the chemical you're exposed to, it's *when* you're exposed. A chemical hitting a fetus at four weeks can be much more harmful than the same dose three months or six months later. Damage from such exposures may not appear for decades, long after the original exposure occurred. It has proven very difficult to assess what kind of damage might occur from exposures to a multitude of chemicals that may interact with each other. After all, no one is ever exposed only to a single chemical, but to many chemicals throughout their lifetime, beginning in the womb.

It was a long and contentious process to get language into this document about the precautionary principle because many countries didn't understand what it meant and were afraid about possibly losing access to useful chemicals. And many countries were concerned about losing political support and foreign aid if they disagreed with the wealthier nations, especially with the United States. However, the Swedes always said—and they were real drivers behind this treaty—that if we know a chemical is persistent and lasts a long time, and we know it's bioaccumulative and ends up in our bodies and stays there, and we know it bioconcentrates and works its way up the food chain, then there's a strong presumption of injury. We don't have to prove toxicity by waiting for science to learn the precise linkages between exposure and health outcome if there is sufficient cause for concern about exposure to a particular chemical.

A main idea of the treaty was that not only would it seek to eliminate these twelve chemicals, but a mechanism should be developed to add further chemicals to the treaty for phaseout and eventual elimination if they could be shown to qualify as POPs. The precautionary principle can be used to identify those chemicals.

Using the precautionary principle to identify additional chemicals means that the UN can take precautionary action before science uncovers the precise mechanisms by which a given chemical causes harm, by carefully evaluating all that is known about a particular chemical and then coming to a decision, with public input, about how this chemical should be dealt with. The UN has set up a process whereby it can examine the very best science regarding chemicals for which there is some concern, including information about their ability to bioaccumulate, to persist, and to travel globally, and then the UN can decide whether such chemicals should be eliminated or severely restricted.

By the final day of negotiations the precautionary principle had been in-corporated into the preamble of the document, which states that the precau-tionary principle needs to be applied to all aspects of implementation of the treaty. The principle is also salted throughout the document.

Vigorous public participation is key, because we all know that it's a mat-ter of politics whether something is considered dangerous or not. How much risk do we want to accept? What do we think the damage is? The public has to be involved in all aspects of the implementation of this treaty. Because these chemicals are potentially harmful at very low levels, when we clean up reser-voirs or contaminated sites, we have to really clean them up, not make a to-ken effort. The public needs to be involved in making sure POPs are removed from products, not created by industrial processes, and that no new POPs are introduced into the marketplace.

There are always splendid ambiguities in treaties, and it's really up to us to keep up the pressure and make sure that our interpretation is enforced. And of course, industry was at all the negotiations in full force, handing the nego-tiators notes, having conversations, taking them out for coffee, lobbying the U.S. delegation at every opportunity. There's always going to be a battle of influence. Industry is always going to be right there to try to come up with its own interpretation of the convention and this interpretation may not protect human and ecosystem health.

It's useful to remember that other countries have already incorporated the precautionary principle into their policies. Sweden is one such country. The Swedes have information that shows that a particular kind of flame retardant is showing up in breast milk in Sweden. This chemical seems to act a lot like PCBs and appears to be both bioaccumulative and persistent. We don't test breast milk in the United States, or haven't for quite some time, although there are isolated studies here and there. The Swedes have been testing breast milk since 1972, and any woman there who wants her breast milk tested can have it done. These women are not any more or less contaminated than anyone else. They give their milk because it's easy to test—it's a little easier to test than fatty tissue or blood. They're giving it so that we all know what's in our bodies.

If this breast milk hadn't been tested, we wouldn't know that flame retardants are probably in all our bodies. Because the Europeans decided the precautionary principle should be used, the European Union is now considering banning these flame retardants from production and use. This is really big news. It's being contested by the manufacturers, who want to keep using a risk assessment model and claim there's insufficient evidence indicating actual harm. The debate is going to go on, and we're at a crisis point. The outcome of the debate will determine whether or not the precautionary principle will begin to become a principle of international law. It's up to us to fight to establish it.

Interestingly, because of all the recent concern about terrorism, our government frequently talks about precautionary measures. If we're talking about precaution in this country, we should also talk about the fact that one out of three zip codes in our country has a chemical facility, either an actual production facility or a water or sewage treatment plant. If it were to be subjected to an accident or terrorist activity, it would spew chemicals within a wide radius. So we're really sitting with a bunch of potential Bhopals in our midst. It makes sense to me that we begin a transition to alternatives, to find cleaner production methods and processes.

We're already raising children at a very difficult time, with a hole in the ozone layer, global warming, the threats of wars and terrorism and new disease vectors, intense environmental crises, and so on. We shouldn't also be bombarding children with disruptive chemicals in the womb and in their most crucial developmental years. Urge your senators to ratify the POPs treaty. Because once we have established a precedent and a firm basis in law for the precautionary principle, we will have a powerful tool with which to begin cleaning up our bodies and our planet.

Part VI

Healing the Spirit

Think Globally, Act Non-locally:
Consciousness beyond Time and Space

Larry Dossey

Dr. Larry Dossey's mind-bending work dissolves the boundaries of what we normally think of as the "environment." He offers the shattering notions that consciousness universally permeates the universe and that consciousness and intention are themselves forces of nature that can be applied to healing.

Larry is a fastidious researcher, and there are wheelbarrows of data to back him up. But this kind of nonlocal healing—nonlocal as in universally and simultaneously ubiquitous—raises many more questions than it answers and has aroused a hornet's nest of opposition. But Larry argues persuasively that the effects of nonlocal consciousness are simply too overwhelming to ignore.

His path to this work has been a winding one. The son of a sharecropper in the cotton fields near Waco in central Texas, he grew up in the buckle of the Bible Belt and spent a lot of Sunday mornings in revival meetings. At the age of sixteen, he was touring Texas with a gospel quartet, playing piano for a fire-and-brimstone tent evangelist and planning to become a preacher. But then he decided college would offer better career choices. He was born again into scientific rationalism and went on to medical school.

After serving as an army surgeon in Vietnam, Larry became an internist in Dallas, until he ran into a big problem. He developed severe migraines that posed a potentially serious threat to his patients. Without any effective standard medical treatments at hand, he decided to try biofeedback. It worked.

The experience launched him on a journey into the realm of mind-body medicine, unearthing an underground of seemingly miraculous recoveries that did not conform to conventional medical materialist models. He didn't forsake the scientific method; in fact, he redoubled his scientific rigor to disprove these mysterious hap-

penings. *He went on to become chief of staff at Medical City Dallas Hospital, until a herniated disc compelled him to give up his practice.*

That was our good luck, since he has gone on to author a series of pathfinding books, including Healing Words *and* Prayer Is Good Medicine, *meticulously documenting the evidence of the power of prayer in healing. He is also the executive editor of the journal* Alternative Therapies in Health and Medicine, *the top peer-reviewed journal in the field of holistic and integrative medicine. He writes elegant essays in each issue that are collected for his latest book,* Healing beyond the Body: Medicine and the Infinite Reach of the Mind. *Larry also served as co-chair of the Panel on Mind/Body Interventions of the Office of Alternative Medicine at the National Institutes of Health. He works closely with his wife, Barbara Dossey.*

The impact of his work has been phenomenal. Before Healing Words *was published in 1993, only three medical schools offered courses in the role of religious practice and prayer in health. Today over eighty medical schools have such courses, many of which use Larry's works as textbooks. He has been a singular force for bringing wholeness and holiness back to medicine and imbuing it with a reverence for the sacred.*

❋   ❋   ❋

ABOUT SIX YEARS AGO there were only three medical schools in the country that would have anything to do with the idea that spirituality had relevancy to human health. But the data that has accumulated since then has been so compelling that now 80 of the 125 medical schools in the country have developed formal courses committed to exploring the associations between spiritual practice, religious devotion, intercessory prayer, and health. The taboo separating spirituality and medicine has been broken.

One of the most controversial and challenging concepts in this whole movement of intercessory prayer is the idea that you could have an empathic, compassionate, loving, prayerful thought for someone at a distance that could have some effect, even if that person might not know you were doing it. A few years ago that was considered outrageous.

The problem that we have faced in trying to bring spirituality back into medicine is that we "know" up front that it's not possible for something like intercessory, distant, off-site prayer to work because the dominant paradigm views the brain's workings, or what we call mind, to be a consequence of its anatomy and its physiology, and nothing more.

Francis Crick, the Nobel-Prize-winning codiscoverer of the structure of DNA, put it this way: "A person's mental activities are entirely due to the behavior of the nerve cells, glial cells and the atoms, ions and molecules that make them and influence them." According to this view, thoughts are equivalent to the brain. They cannot reach out in space and time and possibly make a difference, so we know ahead of time that this stuff can't work. Doctors know. We know these things.

The problem is that the data hasn't gotten the message. There are also other competing points of view that are usually brushed aside. For example, Professor John Searle, one of the most distinguished philosophers in the country, says, "At the present state of the investigation of consciousness, we don't know how it works, and we need to try all kinds of different ideas." Chiming in is Jerry Fodor, another distinguished philosopher in the mind-body area, who says, "Nobody has the slightest idea how anything material could be conscious. Nobody even knows what it would be like to have the slightest idea about how anything material could be conscious. So much for the philosophy of consciousness."

So perhaps consciousness might be able to do things that are unpredictable and that differ from the dogmatic assertions that have dogged us for most of this century. Certain researchers have come forward and have begun to explore the potential operations of consciousness in the world outside the body.

A study was published in 1988 in the *Western Journal Of Medicine* by Fred Sicher, Dr. Elisabeth Targ, and their colleagues at California Pacific Medical Center in San Francisco, which is associated with the University of California at San Francisco School of Medicine. This study looked at the effect of what the researchers called distant intentionality, which included distant intercessory prayer, on the course of patients with advanced AIDS. They did this study twice. In the first version, 40 percent of the unprayed-for group died, and no one in the prayed-for group died. Then they doubled the number of patients and repeated the experiment, looking at related illnesses that kill patients with AIDS, such as pneumocystis pneumonia, meningitis, and so on.

In the repeat study, it looked as if the prayed-for group was receiving some sort of special advantage. They had fewer AIDS-related illnesses. They had to go to the doctor and the hospital less often. When they were hospitalized, their stays were brief. They had a higher level of mental health throughout the study period. In addition, the researchers looked at something that's rarely examined in clinical studies—whether or not the patients believed they were in the prayed-for group. They found that there was no connection between whether the patients *believed* they were receiving prayer and how they did clinically. This finding is important because it shows that you can't explain the results of these studies by saying they are merely the result of positive thinking, expectation, or suggestion—the placebo response.

I phoned Dr. Targ when I heard about this study, because when I learned they were using AIDS patients, my heart sank. I told her over the phone, "Listen, Elisabeth, we don't even have good medical treatment for AIDS, and you're trying to cure AIDS with *prayer* and *distant healing?* Why didn't you pick the flu as your study illness?"

I will never forget her response. She said, "Larry, you are such a weenie. I thought you believed in this stuff." I could see her shaking her finger at me at the other end of the line. She said, "If we can make a difference in AIDS, then the skeptics and the cynics won't be able to come back and say, 'Well, this is an illness they would have recovered from on their own. The people would have gotten better anyway. This doesn't prove anything.' If we can make a difference in AIDS, we've really got something here." And she concluded, "Besides that, there's something else you don't understand. Healers like a challenge."

One of the most high-profile studies in the country is now going on at

Duke University School of Medicine. It is being run by Dr. Mitchell Krucoff, the director of cardiovascular laboratories, and his research associate, a registered nurse and nursing researcher, Suzanne Crater. (In all of these research studies looking at intercessory prayer and healing, there's a nurse behind the scenes.)

This is one of those randomized, double-blind, matched clinical studies. If you were part of this study and you went into Duke University Medical Center's VA hospital for a heart catheterization and angioplasty, a coronary blood vessel dilating procedure, here's what would happen: You would either be being treated conventionally, or you would be treated conventionally and be prayed for. This is a double-blind study; you wouldn't know which group you were in. But if you wound up in the prayed-for group, you would find yourself receiving more prayer overnight that you've probably ever received in your life.

The study organizers notify prayer groups around the globe to begin praying for you. It comes as a virtual shock for these North Carolina patients later to learn about some of the people who were praying for them. For example, the organizers notify, via e-mail, a Buddhist monastery in Nepal to gear up. They notify a monastery in western France to begin to pray. There's even a free intercessory prayer website at www.virtualjerusalem.com. When the site receives notification of a patient's first name and a prayer request, someone writes these on a piece of paper and gives it to a runner, who folds up the paper and slips it into one of the cracks between the stones in the Western Wall in Jerusalem. That is said to give the prayer a special advantage.

The organizers also notify the Silent Unity prayer group in Unity Village, Missouri, part of the Unity Church. They notify many different Protestant churches in the North Carolina area to begin to pray for the Duke patients. One of the most interesting of the assemblies that devote prayers to these patients is a group of nuns cloistered in a convent outside of Baltimore. These nuns just adore praying for these heart patients.

The early data shows this: If patients receive prayer, they have 50 to 100 percent fewer side effects than people who are just treated conventionally in these invasive cardiac procedures. This is what we in this business call "big data." This study was published in the *American Heart Journal* in 2001, the first such study ever published in a professional cardiology journal. The study has been expanded to several other large hospitals around the United States.

I could cite you study after study, not just with cardiovascular disease but with many other diseases. Physicians might want to pay attention to the October 25, 1999, issue of the *Archives of Internal Medicine*, which describes a positive study looking at the effect of intercessory prayer in around a thousand heart patients at St. Luke's Hospital, the Mid-American Heart Institute in Kansas City, Missouri, affiliated with the University of Missouri School of Medicine.

These studies have passed all the tests of what constitutes legitimate science. This field of research is not going to go away. We are literally riding a tidal wave of evidence favoring what I call nonlocal expressions of consciousness.

Let me give you one example of where this field is headed. There was a study done at the Southwest SIDS Center outside of Houston a while back that looked at sudden infant death syndrome (SIDS). The SIDS researchers asked the parents of the babies that had died, "Did you ever have a hunch or a premonition that your child was going to die that was so vivid that you took this concern to your doctor and you made a big deal out of it?" Twenty-one percent of these people said, "Yes, we knew our baby was going to die, and we told the doctor. We made an issue of it." Then the researchers wondered if parents just normally go around having these kinds of fears and anxieties. So they asked parents of normal babies, "Have you ever had this feeling?" Only 2.1 percent of them said yes.

But when the parents who had premonitions took their concerns to the pediatrician and said, "Our baby is going to die. We know it. We've got to do something," in every case, without exception, the doctor responded to the parents with what the researchers called placating denial, ridicule, or outrage. In no instance was the doctor willing to take any further precautions, such as monitoring the baby.

Had these doctors had a worldview of the nature of consciousness that would permit the nonlocal acquisition of information, some of those babies would be alive. These nonlocal manifestations of consciousness seem to indicate the mind's ability to function outside of space and time, to escape the confines of the brain and the body.

I had a patient show up in my office in Dallas. She stuck her head in the office without an appointment one morning and said, "I am scared to death. You've got to help me. Last night I had a dream in which I saw three little white spots on my left ovary, and I'm terrified this may indicate cancer." We did an examination. It was normal. So then I took her back to the radiologist and I said, "Let's do a sonogram and get a picture of this."

This patient made the mistake of telling the radiologist about her dream. He made fun of her. She had her revenge, however, because the radiologist was back in my office about fifteen minutes later, pale as a ghost, saying, "Well, the sonogram did show three little white spots on her left ovary, exactly as she dreamed. But they were benign cysts, not cancer."

This woman was able to acquire exceedingly specific information that could have made the difference between life and death. So what do we want to do with these things? Do we want to call them merely patient stories or anecdotes? Well, it is true they are stories. In medicine there are two ways we deal with a patient story. If you don't like it, you call it an anecdote. If you like it, you call it a case history.

In another incident reported by dream researchers, a nurse carrying a lamp appeared to a patient in her dreams. The nurse was shining the lamp on the patient's left lower leg, as if to show her something. This went on for a year. The woman couldn't make heads or tails of it, until, a year later, she developed a painful osteomyelitis (bone infection) at the specific site where the woman in the dream was holding the light. This is the iconic, archetypal image of Florence Nightingale, the nurse with the lamp, one of the great women in the history of healing.

So how might nonlocality of consciousness work? Most people currently in medical science who pay attention to it are stuck in a classical mechanical image of how they think it might work. Because there are two people involved, the receiver and the healer, most researchers think there's got to be some sort of mechanical, energetic connection between them. In my view this is a dead end. We are going to have to overcome these images that there's some sort of signal between these two people that's somehow explainable by classical manifestations of energy.

Some people have this idea that there's directionality to it, that something is flowing in one direction or another. These images are hopelessly flawed. I think that the image that is going to carry the day is going to be one that is genuinely nonlocal, which overcomes the idea that anything is sent. If you try to interpret the data in terms of the old images of classical physics, it just isn't going to work. We are going to have to move toward a nonlocal conceptualization of consciousness if we're going to be able to integrate and explain the sorts of manifestations we've been talking about.

The quality of nonlocal consciousness we see in these experiments is, in my opinion, indirect evidence for something that genuinely resembles the idea of the soul, something that is immortal, eternal, and omnipresent. The spiritual connotations of a nonlocal theory of consciousness, I believe, are relatively profound.

Skeptics say, "We know the data couldn't be right because you don't have any theories to support it." Actually we are drowning in hypotheses and theories that account for this sort of thing, some being advanced by Nobel Prize winners, such as Brian Josephson. Almost all of the theories have this nonlocal flavor, in which consciousness is freed from the confines of the brain and body and also from the confines of the present moment.

It is said by cynics and skeptics that good scientists don't play this game. Good scientists don't go there. That is a piece of stereotypical nonsense that needs to be discarded. There was a survey that was done fairly recently and published in *Nature*, one of the world's most prestigious science journals, that found that 39 percent of American biologists, mathematicians, and physicists *do* believe in a supreme being who would respond to distant, intercessory prayer.

The boggle threshold is that level in your mind at which you become so antagonized by an idea that you just shut off, and after that the data doesn't matter. There is something about this field of spirituality and the nonlocality of consciousness that makes most scientists and doctors go ballistic. I mention it because if you deal with this in your private life or with your physician or in your community, you're going to bump into it, so I just want to give you a glimpse of how this works.

Ray Hyman is the dean of skeptics, cynics, and critics in this country toward this field. A University of Oregon psychologist, Hyman says the level of the debate in the past 130 years has been an embarrassment for anyone who would like to believe that scholars and scientists adhere to standards of rationality and fair play. He's right. As an example, one scientist wrote in *Science*, perhaps the most prestigious science journal in the world, "Not one thousand experiments with ten million trials and by one hundred separate investigators giving total odds against chance of 1,000 to one could make me accept ESP."

One looks for a term to dignify these kinds of stances. The best one I can come up with is bigotry. Herman von Helmholtz, the most prominent physicist of the nineteenth century, said, "I cannot believe it. Neither the testimony of all the fellows of the Royal Society, nor even the evidence of my own senses would lead me to believe in the transmission of thought from one person to another independently of the recognized channels of sensation. It is clearly impossible."

Here's my favorite quote from a famous skeptic: "This is the sort of thing I wouldn't believe even if it were true." Thus Einstein was led to say, "It's harder to crack a prejudice than an atom." But the skeptics and the cynics are on the run. The only reason eighty medical schools currently have courses in this stuff is because of the evidence, because of the data.

Carl Sagan was no fan of what we've been talking about, but Carl got this right. In his commencement speech at the University of California at Los Angeles in 1991, he said, "It is the responsibility of scientists never to suppress knowledge, no matter how awkward that knowledge is, no matter how it may bother those in power. We are not smart enough to decide which pieces of knowledge are permissible and which are not."

What is the future of integrative medicine? Niels Bohr, one of the patriarchs of modern quantum mechanics, once said that prediction is very difficult, particularly of the future. I think he was right, but I would nonetheless like to take a shot at predicting the future for this field. I would suggest that when any new idea crops up in medicine, it is generally possible to observe a four-step process by which people respond to this new idea. This process has been played out time and time again in the past few decades with regard to how the public and the profession view a new therapy, whatever it happens to be.

First, in conventional medicine, the skeptics almost always say that the new therapy just has no effect. Their predictable phrase is that it is "junk science."

The second stage in the response is that as evidence favoring the new therapy continues to emerge, the skeptics get around to conceding, "Well, what do you know? There is an effect after all. But it's too small to be of any clinical significance."

The third stage is that the skeptics say, "Well, you know, there is an effect, and it's larger than any of us previously thought."

And the fourth stage is when the skeptics say, "We thought of it first."

This is the history of alternative medicine, and I think it's likely to be its future. One of my favorite examples about how this process works is physical exercise, including jogging and running. I'm old enough to recall that thirty years ago the experts said there wasn't any evidence whatsoever that jogging benefited anybody, and people who jogged were called health nuts by physicians.

But over the years the evidence supporting the positive health effects of exercise continued to come forward, and by now, this situation has gone through those four stages that I mentioned. Now we physicians no longer say that jogging is worthless; in fact, we say that it is actually so potent that it's dangerous. You should come into the doctor's office to have a treadmill stress test under a physician's supervision to make sure that it's actually safe for you to engage in this potentially lethal activity. We charge for that, by the way.

So here you have, with regard to something like jogging, all those four stages in action. You have denial, grudging acknowledgment, endorsement, and then claiming the turf as one's own.

As we look to the future of integrative medicine, we ought not to expect all the physicians to come on board, no matter how strong the evidence for any particular therapy proves to be. The fact is that some physicians will simply die off totally unconvinced. There are those physicians out there who are so bitterly opposed to this field that they will be condemning integrative medicine with their final dying breath. But that's one form of change. The famous physicist Max Planck once said that science changes, funeral by funeral. So a new generation of young physicians will arise, and they'll probably look back and wonder what all this fuss was about.

I think the most important development in the future of complementary and alternative or integrative medicine will be a return to something rather radical called healing. What a concept! Here's how I think it may happen.

In the past few years we have bumped up against a factor that I feel is embedded in every therapy that has ever been used by healers or that will be used by healers in the future, and that factor is simply consciousness. In our focus on specific therapies—I don't care whether it's acupuncture, homeopathy, herbs, or nutrition—we have largely, even in the field of integrative and complementary and alternative medicine, managed to pretty much overlook the role of consciousness. When I use this term, I am not talking about things like positive thinking, suggestion, and expectation, what is usually called the placebo response. I am talking about something a good deal more outrageous than that. I'm referring to the power of consciousness to bring about actual changes in the state of the outside physical world, changes that may occur at a distance from the individual in ways that promote wholeness and healing.

There's a recent study on intercessory prayer that was done at Columbia University College of Physicians and Surgeons. It was published in the September 2002 issue of the *Journal of Reproductive Medicine.* The study involved 219 women aged twenty-six to forty-six who were consecutively treated with in vitro fertilization and embryo transfer. That's the procedure in which fertility experts harvest an egg from the ovary, fertilize it in a test tube, then transfer it back to the woman's uterus. Then they keep their fingers crossed, basically, hoping that a successful implantation and pregnancy will result. This was a so-called triple-blind study. That meant that there were two groups— a treatment and a control group—and the patients in them did not know which group they were in, as in a double-blind study, but in addition to that, the health care workers (the doctors and the health care team) did not know that the study was going on. Everybody was totally in the dark about the existence of the experiment.

The women who were in the treatment group and were assigned intercessory prayer had a 50 percent successful pregnancy rate, whereas the women who were not assigned intercessory prayer had a 26 percent pregnancy rate. The likelihood that you could explain this outcome according to chance was on the order of 13 in 10,000.

So how good is the evidence in this field? Not only have there been many persuasive studies, there have been seven meta-analyses or systematic analyses done by professional statisticians. All but one of these systematic or metaanalyses are positive, some of them stunningly positive.

Many studies in nonhumans explore, for example, the healing rates of surgical wounds in animals, the replication rates of bacteria in test tubes, the rapidity of growth of fungi in petri dishes, the germination rates of seeds, the growth rate of seedlings under laboratory conditions, and the specific rate of biochemical reactions in test tubes. These studies are important because you can do them with fanatical precision. They leapfrog almost all of the complaints that skeptics level at the human studies in the field.

These nonhuman studies are important for another reason. If you back off and you look at this field as a whole, what you see is that the nonlocal effects of consciousness operate across an immense spectrum of nature. They are not confined just to the human level. You see these intentionality and prayer effects from the micro or atomic-molecular level through the meso or middle world, where bacteria live, up to the macro world inhabited by humans and plants and animals. This linkage, this so-called concatenation or coming together of effects, unifying these vastly different domains of nature, is one of the most compelling aspects of this field. This sort of concatenation is a highly valued feature of valid science. It suggests that we're dealing with a general principle that is embedded throughout all nature, and that we're not fooling ourselves about the existence of the phenomenon.

These studies involve two main processes: healing and fertility. The healing studies involve the repair of actual wounds and the healing of specific diseases, such as AIDS and coronary artery disease. The fertility studies involve not just the fertility of humans but the fertility of the nonhuman world as well, such as the germination rate of seeds and the growth rates of plants.

I would suggest that these healing and fertility studies ought to function as a wake-up call for the entire eco-environmental movement, because what are we involved in if not the fertility and the healing of the earth?

Some of the world's most recognized scholars who have taken the trouble to explore this data have concluded that something real is happening here. Jessica Utts, an internationally recognized mathematician and statistician at the University of California at Davis, says in referring to the role of consciousness in retrieving information nonlocally, "Using the standards applied to any other area of science, it is concluded that psychic functioning has been well established. Arguments that these results could be due to methodological flaws in the experiments are soundly refuted. The statistical results of the studies are far beyond what is expected by chance. Effects of similar magnitude have been replicated at a number of laboratories across the world, and such consistency cannot be readily explained by criticisms or claims of flaws or fraud. Psychic functioning is reliable enough to be replicated properly in properly conducted experiments with sufficient trials to achieve the long-run statistical results needed for replicability."

We desperately need to recognize the relevance of these kinds of studies to environmentalism. If we don't, we're going to make the same mistake that twentieth-century medicine made when it believed that it was not necessary to make a vital place for the mind in healing. That has not proved possible for medicine, and it's not going to prove possible for the environmental movement.

Alfred North Whitehead once said, "It is no exaggeration to say that the future course of history depends on the decisions made by this generation as to the relationship between science and religion." In the aftermath of September 11th, we need this recognition more than ever. One of the lessons of that day, it seems to me, is that the attempts to force either religion or science into isolation from each other can lead to unspeakable disaster. The secular scientific and the religious sides of life cannot be kept in separate boxes. They *literally* bleed into one another, as we've painfully seen. This is not a new recognition.

Ralph Waldo Emerson said, "The religion that is afraid of science dishonors God and commits suicide." Einstein said, "Science without religion is lame. Religion without science is blind."

But what kind of religion or spirituality is fit to claim our allegiance? The events of September 11th have shown us once again—and we always seem to need to relearn this lesson—that religion can be perverted in utterly grotesque ways, and so we have to be careful in how we wish to see science and religion and spirituality come together. This is not a simple issue. Here is where the evidence for the healing effects of nonlocal mind help us.

You will see that the effects of distant healing and intercessory prayer point like an arrow to religious tolerance and openness, because they clearly show that no particular religion has cornered the market on these phenomena. These effects are universal. There is no monopoly. These studies provide hope for our tortured earth because they show that those old-fashioned ideas of love and empathy and compassion can literally change the state of the physical world in positive ways. Never have people of goodwill needed to employ these effects more than now.

Reading the Mind of Nature:
Ecopsychology and Indigenous Wisdom

Leslie Gray

Leslie Gray has for decades been one of the most creative innovators to blend ancient and modern healing practices. She has evolved a form of "shamanic counseling" (a term she coined) that combines the insights of modern psychology with the time-tested practices of indigenous healing and ceremony.

Of Oneida and Seminole ancestry, she is a psychologist in private practice in San Francisco. She also teaches ecopsychology and Native American studies at several Bay Area universities, including the University of California at Berkeley, the California Institute of Integral Studies, and San Francisco State University. She leads unique travel and study programs to sacred sites in the southwestern United States. A member of the Society of Indian Psychologists and board member of the Association for Transpersonal Psychology, she is founder of the Woodfish Institute, which promotes ecological education grounded in indigenous wisdom.

Leslie knows we will need to draw from the best of the world's ancient wisdom traditions as well as the leading edges of contemporary creativity to begin to heal a wounded civilization. She shows us that, with exquisite attention and intention, we can blend old and new, passion and intellect, to create the psychological and spiritual wholeness that will help us rediscover our place in the web of life.

✿   ✿   ✿

A PARTICULAR WORLDVIEW, model of healing, and system of values underlie our current treatment choices in the field of mental health. But how would we be thinking and what would we be doing if we had a genuinely "ecotherapeutic" model of mental health that portrayed human beings as part of the natural world? I believe the emerging field of ecopsychology offers us such a model and a framework in which to rediscover and re-create very effective ancient healing practices.

The prevailing Euro-American version isn't a model of health; it's a model of illness. That's why so much of our materia medica is "anti"—antibacterial, anti-inflammatory, antidepressant, and so on. The Native American model of health emphasizes restoring balance—aligning body, mind, and heart in balance with the environment—and understands that this is a process: You lose the balance; you regain it. You lose the balance; you regain it. That's why in Pueblo ceremonies, at the most sacred of moments, they send out the clowns to make fun of all the elders and the medicine people there, and indeed of the entire ritual. They resist a naïve notion of "holy." They do not try to get rid of all problems or all evil: They try instead to find nature's balance between positive and negative. That's very different.

The term *koyaanisqatsi*, which means "life out of balance," is now well known because of a popular film, but very few people know how that concept is used in healing. In one Navajo healing ceremony, for example, patients sit on a sand painting throughout what is often a four- to seven-day process to go back through their lives and review them, trying to get from the place of *koyaanisqatsi*, where their life went out of balance, to *hozho nahasdlii*, to harmony restored. The patient is in a *hogan* with friends and family around, harmonious songs are sung, and the patient sits in an exquisitely balanced sand painting, with beautifully carved fetishes placed on various parts of the body. All the imagery suggests harmony restored, a return to balance or health. In

Navajo, the word for balance, the word for harmony, and the word for beauty are the same word: *hozho.*

The Judeo-Christian worldview tells us we have been kicked out of paradise due to our sinful ways and that we must rid ourselves of sin to ascend to paradise. That's a fractured or broken image, and, though science has challenged the church's dogmas, that altruistic model still unconsciously informs Western psychology.

Asian cultures that see existential phenomena as resulting from the interaction of opposites such as yin and yang, and which focus on energy flows in nature and in the body, are informed by a more dynamic and holistic model than the West's, but those cultures have still produced some of the most hierarchical and patriarchal of all societies. Both the European and the Asian models have resulted in hierarchical, patriarchal societies. That, in my view, is because both focus on unity or "paradise" as an abstraction, whereas the indigenous worldview is that this world is already paradise. It's an earth-based spirituality, rather than an attempt to transcend the earth with spirituality.

Through Woodfish Institute, we've been trying to help introduce indigenous approaches to mental health into the mainstream. We funded a researcher to present a paper at the annual American Psychological Association's meeting, a paper on how psychologists and psychiatrists have traditionally misperceived shamans and classified them as schizophrenic. I've also been doing training for the outpatient psychiatric staff at some Kaiser hospitals, as well as for the Japan Institute of Psychotherapy. At Kaiser I set up a medicine wheel, right there in the windowless rooms of their outpatient psychiatric facility. I established north, south, east, and west and got everybody up on their feet, focused on a question, and started drumming. We walked around the wheel and asked questions of the wheel from different perspectives. It's astonishing how quickly the participants' worldviews shifted and how much creativity was released.

A case study from my practice highlights how an indigenous approach to individual therapy can work. I call this case "a dream of a red spider." Jane was a psychotherapist I met when she attended several prayer tobacco circles. Recently divorced and new to the San Francisco Bay Area, she still hadn't found work and was adjusting to living with a new lover. She described herself as depressed. At the prayer smoke, she would cry for most of the two hours. She had a rash on her hands, which a dermatologist had said could not be accounted for medically. The discomfort of the rash only added to her ever-present anxiety. A turning point in my three months of individual work with her occurred after a session in which I restored her guardian spirit. The next night, she had a nightmare in which a red spider attached itself to her vagina. At our next session she asked, "What does it mean?"

She was a psychotherapist, so meaning was important to her. I told her that meaning is only one way of working with dreams. The shamanic way would be for me to remove the spider. She looked baffled but agreed to a ceremony for removing harmful power instrusions. I had her lie down on my office floor, and I sat behind her head with a power object in one hand and a rattle in the other. As I shook my rattle and began to enter a non-ordinary consciousness, I noticed a spider strolling up the pillow on which I was sitting. At first I ignored it, trying to stick to the business at hand, but finally I stopped rattling, picked up the creature, and held it in my open palm. I sat up, Jane sat up, and we looked into my palm. She turned white as a sheet and shrieked. In her dream, she had seen a red spider exactly like the one in my hand, with the same red markings on its back. I picked up the ordinary spider, took it outside, released it, and returned to my original task of removing the non-ordinary spider. After that session, Jane showed dramatic improvement. She reported feeling more energy, and began to go for job interviews and actively pursue new relationships. More important, she no longer described herself as depressed.

I think that to restore our personal and collective sanity we need to get back on track, to rediscover a universe of living beings intimately related: the biosphere as our family. This family has values: respect for life, harmony with nature's cycles, gratitude, balance, and above all, reciprocity—don't take anything without giving something back. This is the key. Reciprocity with Being underlies indigenous cures.

Another project I've begun is the Woodfish Prize. I decided to offer a prize for a Native American and a Euro-American who could work together in a mutually transformative way on a project. At the end of the first year, I had decided not to give the prize. There were about two more days before the deadline was up, and I'd read all the submissions, and I felt no one had really gotten the idea of "mutual." But right at the deadline, I got a perfect example of what I'd been looking for. A professor at a university took a sabbatical and went to the only Native American traditional ground in central California and helped dig a ceremonial ground. He had been at a talk I had given and had heard me mention that frequently people asked me how to meet an authentic Native American shaman. I said that rather than wandering around reservations looking for enlightenment, you might try going and seeing what the people say they actually need and rolling up your sleeves and pitching in. He did so, and it changed him profoundly. He developed a relationship with the elder who is building the ceremonial space that was mutually transformative.

Stopping the War on Mother Earth

Melissa Nelson

Melissa Nelson is an inveterate pollinator. She judiciously distributes bits of cultural DNA between the indigenous and the mainstream, fertilizing the future with the best of both worlds. A member of the Turtle Mountain band of Chippewa, she is a writer, educator, and activist focused above all on the conservation and restoration of indigenous lands and cultures. For the past ten years she has served as executive director of the Cultural Conservancy, a Native American organization dedicated to conserving traditional cultures and their ancestral lands.

Melissa has done remarkable work with the Cultural Conservancy to preserve and document a wide range of threatened Native languages and cultural legacies. She has also supported indigenous groups' efforts to defend their rights and revitalize their communities. Her efforts have led to land-rights victories for California Indians and to invaluable oral histories collected from surviving elders. She is a gifted ambassador and bridge builder, helping establish ties among indigenous communities in places as disparate as Hawaii, Tibet, and California. With her musician-producer husband, Colin Farish, she has nurtured an impressive range of cultural initiatives and collaborations, including the Storyscape project, which has recorded for future generations the stories and storytelling traditions of California Indians.

Melissa keeps one foot in the world of formal education. She holds a doctorate in cultural ecology from the University of California at Davis and has taught ecopsychology at the California Institute of Integral Studies. She is currently a professor in the American Indian Studies Department at San Francisco State University. Of mixed Chippewa, Norwegian, and French ancestry, Melissa is someone who gracefully blends indigenous ways with the rigors of modern intellectual disciplines. Her work perfectly illustrates the wondrous benefits of crosscultural cooperation.

＊　　＊　　＊

IN CALIFORNIA, we are certainly in one of the most biologically diverse areas in the world, but we are also in a cultural diversity hot spot. California had and continues to have a remarkable variety of native peoples. And even though a lot of plant and animal species are tragically becoming extinct, many Native American communities, contrary to popular opinion, are not extinct. The media and history books chronically under-represent the California Indians' presence and population and treat them as invisible. Most people think California Indians are virtually gone. That is a serious misperception. They are still here and there is a lot we can learn from them.

Ecopsychology is an attempt to bring ecology and psychology together again. All traditional peoples know that you cannot have a healthy mind or a healthy community without healthy land and a healthy environment. Oren Lyons, the great Iroquois leader, says, "We will continuously have human wars until we stop our war against Mother Earth." Ecopsychology is about stopping that war on Mother Earth and restoring harmony and balance.

If we truly want to restore the earth and heal our minds and our communities, we have to restore our relationship with the earth that we're standing on, our true mother. Indigenous knowledge can help us do that, but how do we honor ancestral knowledge or ancient wisdom in these postindustrial times? California Indian people have suffered some of the worst genocidal policies any human community has ever suffered through, and yet there are many California Indian communities actively working to bring back their native plants and restore medicines, traditional foods, languages, stories, and songs. Through my work with the Cultural Conservancy, I feel very honored to collaborate with many of these communities.

One project of great interest is in San Diego County. It's called the Tribal Digital Village. San Diego has eighteen Indian reservations, more than any other county in the nation. These groups are working in partnerships with Hewlett-Packard, which provided them with $5 million worth of equipment and technical training. An incredible group of young tribal members are going around talking to their elders, their teachers and wisdom keepers, and recording them on audio- and videotape. They are turning the information into digital stories, films, and CDs. It's a great example of a community healing project that combines the best of ancient wisdom and modern technology to foster the survival of knowledge and culture.

Just as there's a link between biological diversity and cultural diversity, there's a link with psychological diversity. The languages that indigenous people speak reflect completely different ways of thinking that are extremely important to preserve and restore and for us to have access to. Native peoples have worked for thousands of years to maintain a harmonious relationship with the earth. They haven't always succeeded. Indian people are just like all people; we all make mistakes, but long-lasting cultures were often the ones that learned most effectively from those mistakes. That's why they emphasized the natural law of reciprocity. You don't take something without giving something back. That's certainly something that globalized capitalism is not thinking about, and it desperately needs to be reintegrated into our worldview.

All of the world's diverse languages (approximately 6,000 today), whether they're from Europe, Africa, Asia, the Americas, or the Pacific Islands, remind us that there are different ways of thinking, and as Einstein said, "You cannot solve your problems with the same thinking that created your problems." So we need to keep alive and explore these different ways of thinking and being. I, for example, as a mixed-blood Native person, look not only to my own indigenous roots in the Chippewa tradition but also to my European, French, and Norwegian ancestry in order to draw from a wide range of perspectives. We need all the help we can get.

We're living in very dark times, and there are many reasons to get depressed, and yet I find so much hope in these communities that are restoring their knowledge and languages and keeping them alive through modern technology. It's very refreshing. Survival is all about adaptation, and ecopsychology is one useful approach to finding new ways to adapt to an insane world by going back to some of the roots of healing that indigenous people have developed and shared.

Green Medicine and Plant Spirit

Kathleen Harrison

If Kathleen Harrison isn't a real "plant person," no one is. A courageous and profoundly dedicated independent ethnobotanist, she has devoted much of her life to the study of the many-faceted relationship between plants and people. For over twenty-five years she has examined the folk uses of plants in ritual, art, medicine, and food, with a special emphasis on the stories and beliefs that accompany the indigenous appreciation of nature. The focus of her fieldwork has been the cultures of Mexico, Amazonian Peru, Ecuador, and the contemporary herbal and shamanic subcultures of the western United States. Kat teaches widely and writes about the history and traditions of plant use, knowledge, and wisdom with a totally unique voice.

She also is a gifted photographer and illustrator. She teaches the art of perception through classes in botanical illustration and guided walks in nature. She is co-founder and project director of Botanical Dimensions, a modest nonprofit organization that has supported ethnobotanical fieldwork and living plant collections in various countries since 1986. Special funds help support traditional healers and their families, part of an effort to encourage the transmission of their unique knowledge to members of their own communities.

Kat is currently teaching classes at the California School of Herbal Studies and in the Point Reyes Field Seminar program, as well as a course called "Plants in Civilization" at Sonoma State University. Through the Center for Healing and Spirituality affiliated with the University of Minnesota, she leads ethnobotany field courses in Hawaii. Recently she has been writing about her extensive fieldwork with the Mazatec Indians of Mexico and their remarkable visionary prayer ceremonies, which are largely dedicated to healing.

I HAVE WORKED MANY YEARS in the realm of people, plants, and plant medicines. In the 1970s I spent quite a while in the Peruvian Amazon, working with healers who used a spectrum of plants from the most subtle to the most powerful. Then I came back to my life in California and did many other botanical projects. It was only in the early 1990s, when I went back to the Amazon, that I completely "got" the idea of plant spirit. In fact, it was no longer an idea; it became a reality and got under my skin, changing my life substantially.

Since then, I've done quite a lot of fieldwork with Mazatec Indians in the mountains of Oaxaca in Mexico. Little by little, here where I live, I continue to learn about the Native California Indian relationship to nature and plants. I see wonderful parallels among these nature-based societies in which everything is animate and every species is a being. We so-called Westerners also need to develop an intrinsic perception of this hidden reality. One benefit would be to empower the medicine that we grow, that we are given, or that we purchase, making it even more effective.

Since our culture is so reductionist and materialist, it's even more important that we who tend to be intellectual and commercial in our orientation—who recognize matter much more readily than we recognize spirit—learn from models that can help us understand spirit in nature and spirit in medicine.

The word "spirit" comes from the Latin for breath—think of inspiration, respiration—so what we're talking about when we say a plant or a species has a spirit is that it draws energy from the universe and expresses it in a particular form. The ancient notion in many cultures is that there were primordial beings that came before us who were much larger individuals than we all are. They were a different order of being, yet they interacted and had relationships, love affairs, conflicts, and exchanges of all sorts. As history fell into a more profane or complex time, according to some mythologies, each of those beings became a species.

According to that type of ancient belief, which is truly global, we humans, as complex and differentiated as we may seem, are one being, and each of the plant species that we take and use as medicine is also a being. I've learned from my Native friends that we must talk to the spirit of each one of those plants. Whether you're ingesting it or growing it in your garden or passing by it in the forest, you learn to talk to it as though it were a being who, in its genes and in its form, carried a constellation of qualities, actions, and ways of interacting with us; a being whom we need to speak to, not just know about. To know about it is a step. To speak to it is really what makes the medicine work. That is the relationship: to speak to it, to listen to it.

These concepts are rooted in the way that Native people—those people who are still close to the earth around the world—live their daily lives. Let's remember that there are some really basic principles, and one of the most basic in relating to the natural world is reciprocity.

When, for instance, you meet a plant and you wish to take some of its body for medicine, you ask it if you might, and you explain what it's for, and you give it something back. On this continent it often has been tobacco, traditionally the most sacred plant of the Americas, that is offered in exchange. I've thought about what is most valuable to people of our contemporary culture, and I think it's *time*. Time is the thing that is most expensive to us, what we have the least of, and what we're the most jealous with. Time is the precious gift that we can offer to a plant if we want to get to know it, when we want to ask something from it. The way we can offer it time is to get to know the plant, sit with it, learn what it looks like, and maybe grow it. Even if you're just purchasing the dried root, try to learn about that plant's world.

That's what you're communicating with: the character of the species within its own worldview. The medicine really is coming through the whole chain of the experience of that species in evolution. Recently, I've used the herbal medicine called goldenseal, and so I've been thinking more than usual about it. Goldenseal is native to the moist forests and meadows of eastern

North America. Its root is what we use for medicinal purposes. Its core is brilliant yellow, a golden root, and it often lives through hard winters. In the fall the leaves drop from the small herbaceous plant and its root hunkers down to make it through another season. It has a life experience that it has gathered over eons and eons that comes into the medicine. It's not just another indistinguishable brown powder in a capsule. It's actually one of the species most prized as medicine in Native America. It's also a mostly wild species that has been overharvested in recent years, so that now goldenseal has to be protected and is being replanted in its own native woodlands. Now is the time for humans to return that gift we've been so eagerly harvesting in recent decades.

I also like to learn a plant's chemistry when I can, as part of this relationship. For instance, it can be helpful to know that hydrastine, which is a chemical in goldenseal, swells and explodes the cells of bacteria that it meets in our bodies. That's how it does the job, which is amazing in itself, but I think that we tend to look for those operational reasons and then we forget that spirit is at work there too. I have heard it said that a species of plant is actually a spirit that has chosen to be dressed in the form that you witness. That form is the exquisite gown it has put on, and that is the medium that we're collecting when we're asking the spirit to be active in our bodies.

So when you take goldenseal because you think you're getting a sore throat, you speak to it, because you've learned something about this plant and you've given it your time. You speak to it, even when taking the tea or the tincture, and ask, "Who are you?" Then listen and ask, "Would you be willing to help me? Would you be my ally?" And then, "What would you like? What can I do for you?" It may not be something that would be an apparent, obvious exchange, perhaps just a heartfelt, murmured "Thank you." Yet it creates a kind of receptivity to the plant's qualities. We need to remember to be receptive and reciprocal in order to understand what herbalism, green medicine, really is about.

So medicine, in the traditions I've worked in, is not just about chemistry. It's about that which heals. Many cultures talk about the songs that come through the plants. If you listen well to a plant whose medicinal aid you have solicited, and give it time, you may be lucky enough to learn its song. Then its song will be as effective a medicine as the plant material itself. That's possible when you've taken that plant in as your deep ally, when you can invoke its medicine without even necessarily touching or finding the plant. It's the spirit of the medicine.

It has been part of my work to go to cultures that use the sacred visionary plants, in Mexico, Ecuador, and Peru. I go to learn their botanical mythology and sometimes their ceremonies involving these plants. These sacramental species have to be met with total respect. Whether they are invoked in ceremony, contemplation, or revelry, these species are powerful beings, and we need to keep that in mind. Like everything else in our culture, even these sacred plants become commodities. The commodification of spirit is really dangerous territory. As individuals, we're not generally wise enough and open-hearted enough to take visionary medicine on our own, or for so-called casual use, without first learning from a teacher or a healer how to engage with such a powerful force. But I can certainly grow a beautiful little peyote plant in a pot of sacred objects, and it's a teacher for me, just by my watching it flower and being near it as a guardian.

A tiny, delicate plant can have a very powerful spirit. A plant's form and stature are not necessarily related to its power. For example, there is a humble, floppy little fungus that grows on wet wood in the Peruvian Amazon. The people appreciate its hydrophilic nature, the way it holds water even when the air is dry, and they use it for food as well as for medicine. On one trip, I'd been in the Amazon for a week but hadn't yet acclimatized to the 90 percent humidity and 90 degree weather, so I was really thirsty and sweating all the time. The people that I was learning from cooked up a little of this fungus in a banana leaf, with a few grains of salt on it. They said, "It's too difficult to boil enough clean water to satisfy your thirst, so eat this." Within an hour my excessive thirst was gone, and for the rest of my long stay I wasn't troubled by it. That's medicine!

Our culture has a strange love-hate relationship with plants, especially those that affect the mind or adjust our energy levels. For example, it is so interesting that finally, after a very long time of denouncing cannabis, we've opened the dialogue enough to talk about it again as medicine. That is what it has been for thousands of years, to many people. After so many years of marginalizing it in the twentieth century, positive studies have finally begun to slip into the discussion. A recent study concluded that marijuana actually relieves pain and that there are an uncanny number of receptors for it in the human body. When used with intention, gratitude, and awareness, it can be a multifaceted medicine. This age-old herb is our sister and ally in many ways, and gradually the tilt of the popular discussion is changing.

I try to keep my eye on the big picture and observe how cultures vacillate in their appreciation and rejection of powerful plants. Fear and denunciation of a species cycle around again to appreciation. We're in a time of such fierce denunciation of tobacco right now that we find it very hard to talk about its holy and sacramental properties. The question is not about the plant being an evil plant or a good plant. It's about how we use it and how conscious we are, and that's true of all medicine.

Unconscious use of anything is damaging, and truly conscious use of anything can make it beneficial, and this goes for food and all the other substances that we love and hate. We seem to go through periods of demonizing the aspects of nature that we don't understand.

Chocolate is another fascinating plant, one that plays multiple roles. Chocolate pods are filled with seeds that have been used as offerings to the gods, and still are. People in Mexico give big dried beans of cocoa to the Virgin Mary; they give them to the spirit of the mountain; and they bring other plants and seeds too. That's what they give as offerings to the gods: plants and seeds. They give them ones that they know will please them. They burn some plants as incense, and some they just lay in sacred places, where water wells up out of the ground.

What you bring as an offering may not necessarily be flowers or spectacular looking things, but very subtle ones. You bring nature to nature, and you bring it as a gift because it shows that you have paid attention and you understand this concept of reciprocity. You don't take from nature without giving something, and then you're always grateful for what you get. That's medicine.

Ecological Medicine:
A Call for Inquiry and Action

From a meeting at Commonweal, Bolinas, California, February 2002. Statement issued September 2002 by the Science and Environmental Health Network. Reproduced Courtesy of SEHN.

Ecological Medicine is a new field of inquiry and action to reconcile the care and health of ecosystems, populations, communities, and individuals.

The health of Earth's ecosystem is the foundation of all health. Human impact in the form of population pressure, resource abuse, economic self-interest, and inappropriate technologies is rapidly degrading the environment. This impact, in turn, is creating new patterns of human and ecosystem poverty and disease. The tension among ecosystem health, public health, and individual health is reaching a breaking point at the beginning of the Twenty-First Century.

Public health measures, education, and medical advances have significantly reduced death and disease in many parts of the world, but some advances come at considerable cost, and the benefits are not equally distributed. Public health systems charged with creating healthful conditions for all have suffered in competition with technologically intensive health care aimed at individual consumers. Health care systems struggle to keep up with the changing patterns of disease that result both from a rapidly changing and degraded Earth and from the way people live. New and old diseases spread with increasing speed within and across national borders. Meanwhile, industrially based medicines and technologies that heal also contribute to the growing burden of environmental toxins in people, air, water, fish, animals, and plants.

Healing disciplines and movements of public health, ecology, conventional medicine, complementary and alternative medicines, conservation medicine, conservation biology, and campaigns such as Health Care Without Harm have sought to address this cycle of conflict among individual health, public health, and ecosystem health in different ways. Ecological Medicine honors these contributions and builds upon them. Ecological Medicine invites the biomedical community, ecologists, scientists, activists, and individuals who are concerned for personal health as well as the health of communities and future generations to learn from each other and to embrace a balanced, ecological approach to sustaining health.

Ecological Medicine integrates the following concepts and values:

- *Interdependence.* Each of us is deeply connected with Earth's ecosystems; each of our lives is only a moment in the grand scale of time. Ultimately, we all depend on the health of the global community and of Earth's biosphere for our own health and happiness. Individuals cannot live healthy or happy lives in poisoned ecosystems and unhealthy communities. By the same token, healthy communities and biological systems depend on human restraint and responsibility in technologies, population, production, and consumption.

- *Resilience.* Health in humans and ecosystems is not a steady state but a dynamic one marked by resilience. Both medicine and ecosystem science and management should focus on promoting and restoring the innate ability of biological systems to protect themselves, recover, and heal. Systems that draw upon or mimic the elegance, economies, and resilience of nature offer promising paths for health care research and development.

- *"First, do no harm."* Health care should not undermine public health or the environment. This precautionary principle should be applied to decisions affecting the ecosystem, populations, communities, and individuals.

- *Appropriateness.* "Medicine," in its Greek origins, means "appropriate measures." The goal is to achieve maximal health with minimal intervention, promoting good health that is appropriate to an individual's stage of life without overburdening Earth's life-sustaining processes.

- *Diversity.* Health is served by diverse approaches, including many traditional healing systems, local adaptations, and indigenous science around the world. Ecological Medicine encourages freedom of medical choice, guided by informed consent and compassionate practice.

- *Cooperation.* In order to gain knowledge and improve practices, patients should be partners with practitioners, and medical professionals should cooperate with ecologists and other students of the natural world. Health care organizations should be managed with the active participation of the communities they serve, while communities must learn to integrate their welfare with that of their regional ecosystems.

- *Reconciliation.* Individual health care services should be economically sustainable, equitable, modest in scale, of high quality, noncommercial, and readily available to all. Societies should build and maintain infrastructures that assure all citizens the capability to meet basic needs such as health, nutrition, family planning, shelter, and meaningful work while minimizing harm to the Earth. Societies should increasingly devote their material and creative resources to policies and projects that restore and maintain the health of biological and human neighborhoods. All efforts to improve human welfare must be conducted with a cooperative framework established by the health of the Earth.

Ecological Medicine sounds an urgent call to action. Understanding the ominous changes in the biosphere compels us to act, individually and collectively. Whether it is in the way we build clinics and hospitals; make, grow, and use medicines; choose areas for scientific study; communicate across disciplines; conduct public health services globally and in particular communities; or choose the means of maintaining our own health, we must do so with a commitment to enhancing life on this planet.

Resources

Part I. Ecological Medicine

Organizations and Websites

The Collaborative on Health and the
Environment
c/o Commonweal
P.O. Box 316, Bolinas, CA 94924
415-868-0970
www.cheforhealth.org
info@cheforhealth.org
Organization committed to reducing public
exposure to environmental toxicants

Collective Heritage Institute / Bioneers
901 W. San Mateo Rd., Ste. L
Santa Fe, NM 87505
877-BIONEER, 877-246-6337
www.bioneers.org
info@bioneers.org

Health Care without Harm
1755 S St. NW, Ste. 6B
Washington, DC 20009
202-234-0091/ Fax: 202-234-9121
www.hcwh.org
info@hcwh.org

Science and Environmental Health Network
3704 W. Lincoln Way, #282
Ames, IA 50014
www.sehn.org

Second Nature
P.O. Box 120007, Boston, MA 02112-0007
www.secondnature.org

Books

Ausubel, Kenny. *The Bioneers: A Declaration
of Interdependence.* White River Junction, VT:
Chelsea Green, 2001 (1997).

Benyus, Janine M. *Biomimicry: Innovation
Inspired by Nature.* New York: William
Morrow, 1997.

Lerner, Michael. *Choices in Healing: Integrating
the Best of Conventional and Complementary
Approaches to Cancer.* Cambridge, MA: MIT
Press, 1994.

Schettler, Ted. *In Harm's Way: Toxic Threats to
Child Development.* Collingdale, PA: DIANE,
2001.

Schettler, Ted, et al. *Generations at Risk:
Reproductive Health and the Environment.*
Cambridge, MA: MIT Press, 2000.

Articles and Periodicals

Brody, Charlotte. "Nurses Can Lead the Charge for Safer IV Bags." March/April 1999. http://www.nursingworld.org/tan/99marapr/asiseeit.htm

Cortese, A.D. "The Role of Engineers in Creating an Environmentally Sustainable Future." *Civil Engineering Practice,* Spring/Summer 1999: 29—38.

Cortese, A.D., and W. McDonough. "Education for Sustainability: Accelerating the Transition to Sustainability through Higher Education." *Environmental Grantmakers Association News and Updates,* Spring 2001: 11—14.

Part II. The "Duh" Principle

Organizations and Websites

Environmental Research Foundation
P.O. Box 5036, Annapolis, MD 21403-7036
888-2RACHEL, 410-263-1584
www.rachel.org
erf@rachel.org

Pesticide Action Network North America
49 Powell St., Ste. 500
San Francisco, CA 94102
415-981-1771
www.panna.org

Physicians for Social Responsibility
1101 14th St. NW, #700
Washington, DC 20005
202-898-0150
www.psr.org
psrnatl@psr.org

Books

Myers, Nancy J. *Ultimate Security: The Environmental Basis of Political Stability.* New York: W.W. Norton, 1994.

Myers, Nancy J., and Norman Myers. *A Wealth of Wild Species: Storehouse for Human Welfare.* Boulder, CO: Westview, 1983.

————, eds. *Gaia, an Atlas of Planet Management.* Garden City, NY: Doubleday Books, 1984.

O'Brien, Mary. *Making Better Environmental Decisions: An Alternative to Risk Assessment.* Cambridge, MA: MIT Press, 2000.

Raffensperger, Carolyn, and Joel Tickner, eds. *Protecting Public Health and the Environment: Implementing the Precautionary Principle.* Washington, DC: Island Press, 1999.

Articles and Periodicals

Rachel's Environment and Health News
Environmental Research Foundation
P.O. Box 5036, Annapolis, MD 21403-7036
www.rachel.org/bulletin/index.cfm?St-1

Raffensperger, Carolyn, and Nancy Myers.
"A Precaution Primer." *YES!* no. 19 (Fall 2001).
http://www.futurenet.org/19technology/
raffensberger.htm

Part III. Public Health, Cancer, and Prevention

Organizations and Websites

American Holistic Nurses' Association
P.O. Box 2130, Flagstaff, AZ 86003-2130
800-278-2462
www.ahna.org

Campaign for Food Safety and Organic
Consumers Association
860 Highway 61, Little Marais, MN 55614
218-226-4164
www.organicconsumers.org

Cancer Prevention Coalition
c/o University of Illinois at Chicago
School of Public Health
2121 W. Taylor St., Chicago, IL 60612
312-996-2297
www.preventcancer.com

Nightingale Institute for Health
and the Environment
P.O. Box 412, Burlington, VT 05402
802-846-1680, fax 802-846-1681
www.nihe.org

Wellspring Media
419 Park Ave. S., New York, NY 10016
212-686-6777
www.wellspring.com
Distributor of the video *Hoxsey: How Healing
Becomes a Crime*, award-winning feature-length
documentary written and directed by Kenny
Ausubel, Realidad Productions, 1987

Books

Ausubel, Kenny. *When Healing Becomes a
Crime.* Rochester, VT: Healing Arts Press,
2000.

Dossey, Barbara Montgomery. *Florence
Nightingale: Mystic, Visionary, Healer.*
Springhouse, PA: Springhouse, 2000.

Dossey, Barbara Montgomery, D.M. Beck,
and L. Selanders. *Florence Nightingale's
Blueprint for Postmodern Nursing: Caring,
Healing, and Spirituality* (in press 2003).

Dossey, Barbara Montgomery, ed. *American
Holistic Nurses' Association Core Curriculum
for Holistic Nursing.* Gaithersburg, MD:
Aspen, 1997.

Epstein, Samuel S. *The Politics of Cancer
Revisited.* Fremont Center, NY: East Ridge
Press, 1998.

Epstein, Samuel S., Lester O. Brown,
and Carl Pope. *Hazardous Waste in America.*
San Francisco: Sierra Club Books, 1982.

Epstein, Samuel S., Suzanne Levert,
and David Steinman. *The Breast Cancer
Prevention Program.* New York: Macmillan,
1997.

Part IV. Nature, Culture, and Medicine

Organizations and Websites

The American Botanical Council
6200 Manor Rd., Austin, TX 78723
512-926-4900, fax 512-926-2345
www.herbalgram.org
abc@herbalgram.org

United Plant Savers
P.O. Box 77, Guysville, OH 45735
www.unitedplantsavers.org
info@unitedplantsavers.org

Ask Dr. Weil
www.drweil.com
A searchable database of health information
and a practitioner referral directory

Books

Achterberg, Jeanne. *Imagery in Healing: Shamanism and Modern Medicine.* Boston: Shambhala, 2002.

————. *Lightning at the Gate: A Visionary Journey of Healing.* Boston: Shambhala, 2002.

————. *Woman as Healer.* Boston: Shambhala, 1991.

Hobbs, Christopher. *Herbal Remedies for Dummies.* Foster City, CA: IDG Books Worldwide, 1998.

————. *Natural Liver Therapy: Herbs and Other Natural Remedies for a Healthy Liver.* Capitola, CA: Botanica Press, 1993 (1986).

Hobbs, Christopher, and Steven Foster. *A Field Guide to Western Medicinal Plants and Herbs.* Boston: Houghton Mifflin, 2002.

O'Mara, Peggy, with Jane McConnell. *Natural Family Living.* New York: Pocket Books, 2000.

O'Mara, Peggy, with Wendy Ponte. *Having a Baby, Naturally.* New York: Atria Books, 2003.

Weil, Andrew. *Eight Weeks to Optimum Health.* New York: Knopf, 1997.

————. *Natural Health, Natural Medicine: A Comprehensive Manual for Wellness and Self-Care.* Boston: Houghton Mifflin, 1990.

————. *Spontaneous Healing: How to Discover and Enhance Your Body's Natural Ability to Maintain and Heal Itself.* New York: Fawcett Books, 1996.

Articles and Periodicals

Alternative Therapies in Health and Medicine
c/o InnoVision Communications, LLC
169 Saxony Road, Ste. 104
Encinitas, CA 92024
866-828-2962
www.alternative-therapies.com

Dr. Andrew Weil's Self Healing Newsletter
P.O. Box 2057, Marion, OH 43305
800-523-3296
www.drweilselfhealing.com

HerbalGram
6200 Manor Rd., Austin, TX 78723
512-926-4900, 800-373-7105
www.herbalgram.org
Journal of the American Botanical Council

Mothering
P.O. Box 1690, Santa Fe, NM 87504
505-984-8116
www.mothering.com
info@mothering.com

Part V. Taking Action

Organizations and Websites

Center for Environmental Literacy
Talcott Greenhouse
Mt. Holyoke College
South Hadley, MA 01075
413-538-3091
www.mtholyoke.edu/proj/cel/

Greenpeace USA
www.greenpeaceusa.org

Iewirokwas Program
www.nativemidwifery.com
Community- and culture-based midwifery
education and practical woman-centered family
birth program

Indigenous Environmental Network
www.ienearth.org

Project Underground
www.moles.org
Vehicle through which environmental, human
rights, and indigenous rights movements can
carry out focused campaigns against abusive
extractive resource activity

UnReasonable Women for the Earth
c/o Collective Heritage Institute / Bioneers
901 W. San Mateo Rd., Ste. L
Santa Fe, NM 87505
877-BIONEER, 877-246-6337
www.bioneers.org

Part VI. Healing the Spirit

Organizations and Websites

Botanical Dimensions
P.O. Box 807, Occidental CA 95465

The Cultural Conservancy
P.O. Box 29044, San Francisco, CA 94129
415-561-6594, fax 415-561-6482
www.nativeland.org
tcc@nativeland.org

Terralingua
1630 Connecticut Ave. NW, Ste. 300
Washington, DC 20009
202-518-2040
www.terralingua.org
info@terralingua.org
Partnership for linguistic and biological
diversity

Woodfish Institute
P.O. Box 29044, The Presidio of San Francisco
San Francisco, CA 94129-0030
415-263-0423
www.woodfish.org

Books

Dossey, Larry. *Healing beyond the Body: Medicine and the Infinite Reach of the Mind.* Boston: Shambhala, 2001.

———. *Prayer Is Good Medicine: How to Reap the Healing Benefits of Prayer.* San Francisco: HarperSanFrancisco, 1996.

———. *Reinventing Medicine: Beyond Mind-Body to a New Era of Healing.* San Francisco: HarperSanFrancisco, 1999.

Roszak, Theodore, Mary E. Gomes, and Allen D. Kanner, eds. *Ecopsychology: Restoring the Earth, Healing the Mind.* San Francisco: Sierra Club Books, 1995.

Articles and Periodicals

Nelson, Melissa. "A Psychological Impact Report for the Environmental Movement." *ReVision* 20, no. 4 (Spring 1998): 37—43.

———, ed. "Introduction to Indigenous Language Revitalization." *ReVision* 25, no. 2 (Fall 2002): 3—5.

Shiva, Vandana. "Monocultures of the Mind." *Trumpeter* 10, no. 4 (1993).

About the Bioneers
and Collective Heritage Institute

Since 1990, Kenny Ausubel and Nina Simons have been assembling the Bioneers for an annual conference, a gathering of scientific and social innovators who have demonstrated model practices and practical models for restoring the earth. These pragmatic strategies effectively address many of our most pressing ecological and societal challenges. Above all, the Bioneers network reflects a culture of solutions.

The Bioneers are biological pioneers who are working with nature to help nature heal and heal ourselves with it. They have peered deep into the heart of living systems to devise strategies for restoration based on nature's own operating instructions. They herald a dawning age of biology founded in natural principles of kinship, interdependence, cooperation, and community.

The Bioneers come from many diverse cultures and perspectives and from all walks of life. They are scientists and artists, gardeners and economists, activists and public servants, architects and ecologists, farmers and journalists, priests and shamans, policymakers and everyday people committed to preserving and supporting the future of life on earth. Uniting nature, culture, and spirit, their visionary and practical solutions also embody a change of heart, a spiritual connection with the fullness of all life that is grounded in social justice.

The stories of the Bioneers demonstrate that just as people have created the environmental and social problems we face, people can also solve them, through a reciprocal partnership with nature. Over and over, their stories show how great a difference the actions of one individual can make.

The Bioneers Conference, a project of the not-for-profit Collective Heritage Institute (CHI), is a "big tent" under which people from many disparate yet related fields gather. The gathering cross-pollinates both issues and net-

ADD 3543

works and serves as a fulcrum for networking and cutting-edge ideas, resources, and connections. The conference has spawned several other projects:

- The Bioneers website offers a rich source of accessible information and connections to numerous other key groups and individuals working for ecological restoration and social justice.

- The radio series *Bioneers: Revolution from the Heart of Nature* each year airs thirteen half-hour programs free to public radio stations across the country and around the world. In 2002 and 2003, the series won the prestigious WorldMedal from the New York Festivals of International Radio and in 2002 was a finalist for the United Nations Department of Public Information Award for programming excellence.

- "Beaming Bioneers" broadcasts live portions of the Bioneers Conference to partner sites as a focal point around which they organize their own mini-conferences, which address local issues and enhance community organizing efforts.

- *The Bioneers Letter*, a biannual newsletter for members of Bioneers/CHI, features articles, program updates, and a calendar and networking section.

- The Bioneers Youth Initiative integrates young people into the Bioneers Conference and helps build connectivity among young activists year-round.

- The Restorative Development Initiative, CHI's Food and Farming program, presents several yearly "Wisdom at the End of a Hoe" training workshops to equip farmers and gardeners with state-of-the-art knowledge on advanced organic growing methods from top practitioners. The program also works with Native American and African American growers on economic development through organic and ecological farming methods.

For more information about the Bioneers and CHI, and to become a member, please contact www.bioneers.org or call toll-free 1-877-BIONEER.